Strength from Within

SURVIVING CANCER: THE POWER OF GIFTS AND HOPE

KIM NELSON

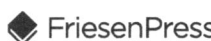 FriesenPress

One Printers Way
Altona, MB R0G 0B0
Canada

www.friesenpress.com

Copyright © 2024 by Kim Nelson
First Edition — 2024

Michelle Peach
Illustrator

ISBN
978-1-03-919705-3 (Hardcover)
978-1-03-919704-6 (Paperback)
978-1-03-919706-0 (eBook)

1. BIOGRAPHY & AUTOBIOGRAPHY, PERSONAL MEMOIRS

Distributed to the trade by The Ingram Book Company

For Kevin,

who held my hand,

wiped my tears,

comforted me,

and gave me strength,

whose love held me up,

gave me hope and courage,

and sat with me every step of the way

to fight my biggest battle.

With immense love, I am eternally grateful to call you my best friend and husband.

TABLE OF CONTENTS

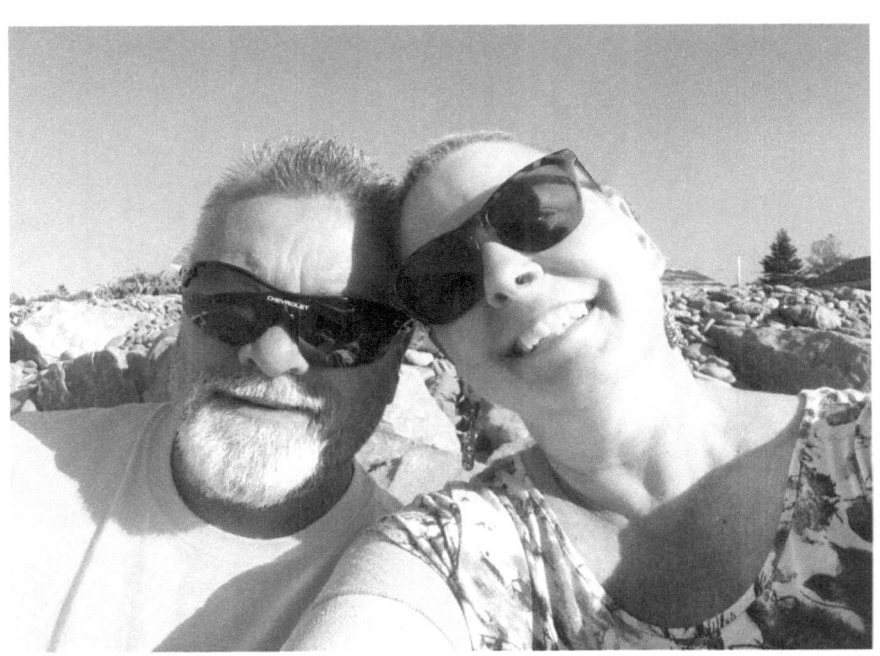

INTRODUCTION

On February 9th, 1963, a baby girl was born in Trenton, Ontario. She would be named Kimberly Anne, daughter to Ron and Gloria and little sister to Mark. My first memory of our home in Trenton, Ontario is of a white, one-level, cottage-style house with a view of beautiful, pristine blue water, which could be seen from the living room window.

My dad was in the military and spent his first posting in Portage la Prairie, Manitoba where my brother, Mark, was born in 1960. My father was posted to Trenton, Ontario, where I joined the family. We lived in Trenton for six years, then in 1969 our family was posted to Cold Lake, Alberta, where we lived for four years. Our next move was a posting to Oromocto, New Brunswick, where we lived for five years—the longest I had ever spent in one location.

We arrived in Oromocto in April 1973; I was nervous to join a class that had already been together since September. I became the new student in the Grade 4 class and luckily made many great friends over the next three months until summer vacation arrived. Our stay provided me the opportunity to complete grades 5 through 9 with my friends.

At the end of Grade 9, I had a great circle of friends and was excitedly awaiting high school in September. Then I learned my dad had been posted. We would be moving to Greenwood, Nova Scotia in August of 1978. I was not thrilled—to say the least.

When we left, my brother drove our older car with me as the passenger, and my mom and dad drove the new burgundy-colored

Dodge Magnum purchased earlier that year. I was filled with sadness as we drove away from Oromocto.

The first year living in Greenwood presented many challenges for me. When opportunities arose, my brother and I would go to visit our friends in Oromocto. Our father drove us to Digby, a ninety-minute drive from Greenwood. We would catch a ferry, which took us to St. John. Our friends would meet us in St. John, and we would drive another hour to arrive in Oromocto. As the first year passed, my friend group dispersed, and my desire to go back to visit began to diminish. I was beginning to make new friends in Greenwood, and I decided to focus my time, energy, and attention on accepting my new surroundings and new friends.

One of my friends from Oromocto, Mary, had moved to PEI, where she met good friends. One of Mary's friends from PEI, Terri, moved to Greenwood. Mary suggested I introduce myself to Terri. I recall being nervous, but I walked over to Terri's house and introduced myself. Terri and I became friends and spent the summer together.

I was fortunate to meet great friends during my high school years. After high school, I attended Annapolis Regional Vocational School in Middleton where I was enrolled in the secretarial program. I enjoyed my year, especially since three of my dear friends—Cricket, Cathy, and Shannon—were enrolled in the same program. After I completed my program, I worked as a secretary on the military base in Greenwood for a year before moving to Winnipeg, where I found a job as a secretary at an advertising agency. I lived in Winnipeg for two years, then ended up in Quesnel, British Columbia. When I lived in Winnipeg, my brother was accepted into the RCMP academy in Regina, Saskatchewan. Mark graduated from the academy in September 1985. I met one of his troop mates during his graduation. We kept in touch with one another and would eventually become a couple. I moved to Quesnel, British Columbia, where he was stationed, and we would marry in late August 1988. Quesnel was a beautiful area, where I met incredible people who to this day hold a special place in my heart. And it was there that I would receive the best gift of my life: my son, James.

When my son was thirteen months old, I moved back to Greenwood. My mom and dad opened their hearts and their home for the two of us to join them. At the age of twenty-eight, my marriage dissolved, and I found myself re-evaluating my life.

At twenty-nine, I decided to attend university and become a teacher. On a sunny September day, I drove to Wolfville to attend Acadia University. I parked my car then began walking up the steep hill to attend my first class. I was petrified. I listened to others around me talking as I walked to the Beverage Arts Centre, BAC. I stopped in front of University Hall contemplating whether I should go to class or go back to the car. Eventually I opted to go to class, and I am forever grateful for making that decision because it started me on path to a career I absolutely love. I was a substitute teacher, then worked as a resource teacher before becoming a school counsellor, a position that has brought me joy, struggles, and great fulfillment.

My life path has had twists, turns, curves, ups, and downs, along with happiness, sadness, fear, loss, and elation. As years have passed, I have adapted to change and displayed my strength and resiliency. The most difficult of all my struggles began on September 5th, 2018, when I learned I had breast cancer.

THE JOURNEY BEGINS

In May 2018, I prepared to complete my exercise routine. I stood in the dining room, feet shoulder-width apart and began hoisting my kettlebell. I squatted with the kettlebell between my legs then moved upward with both hands, to shoulder level. My right arm grazed against my right breast, and I felt "something" protruding toward my bicep. When I examined it with my fingers, I reaffirmed that there was "something." It was hard and sore, but I thought it was muscular, so I did not give it much thought.

A few weeks passed, and I again felt "something" with my arm while exercising, so I asked my husband to feel my breast. He said, "You should get that looked at." I knew he was right, so I made the call to the mobile mammogram bus to make an appointment. Over the phone, they informed me that I could not book an appointment because I had just had a mammogram in October 2017. I could only book an appointment if my last mammogram had been two years ago, so I was instructed to call my family doctor. Our family doctor is located in Mineville, NS, which is an hour and a half away.

I had good intentions to call my family doctor to book an appointment. I work as a school counsellor, and the month of June is always hectic. I was engrossed in getting final reports completed, counselling students, and cleaning my office space. I forgot to call my doctor. When I finally remembered, I was luckily able to book an appointment for June 26th.

Kevin and I arrived in Mineville, sat in the waiting room for a short period of time, then I was called into the exam room.

Dr. Siva asked me to sit on the table. He then pulled my bra away from my breast, felt the area and said, "Yes, that is a lump." He explained the next steps now that the lump had been identified and located. First, I would have a mammogram, and if further investigation was necessary, I would need an ultrasound. The final step would be to have a needle biopsy.

I distinctly remember getting in the truck with Kevin and starting to cry. I said, "Why did he call it a lump?"

Kevin reassured me with his comforting words, "Kim, it's going to be okay." "Let's just wait and get the results from your mammogram." On July 3rd, I went for my mammogram, and on July 6th, I learned further investigation was warranted.

Our son was getting married on July 20th, 2018, and I wanted to focus on this beautiful event in his life, so I did not share my news with anyone except Kevin. At this point, I honestly did not think my lump was harmful, so there was no point in sharing the information with family or friends.

James and Bella arrived from China a few days before the wedding. We were busy finishing the last-minute details. On a hot, sunny Friday afternoon, we watched our James marry the love of his life, Bella. Our dear friend, Lynn, allowed us to have the wedding on her beautiful cottage property in Clementsport. It was truly a magical day with lots of love and laughter.

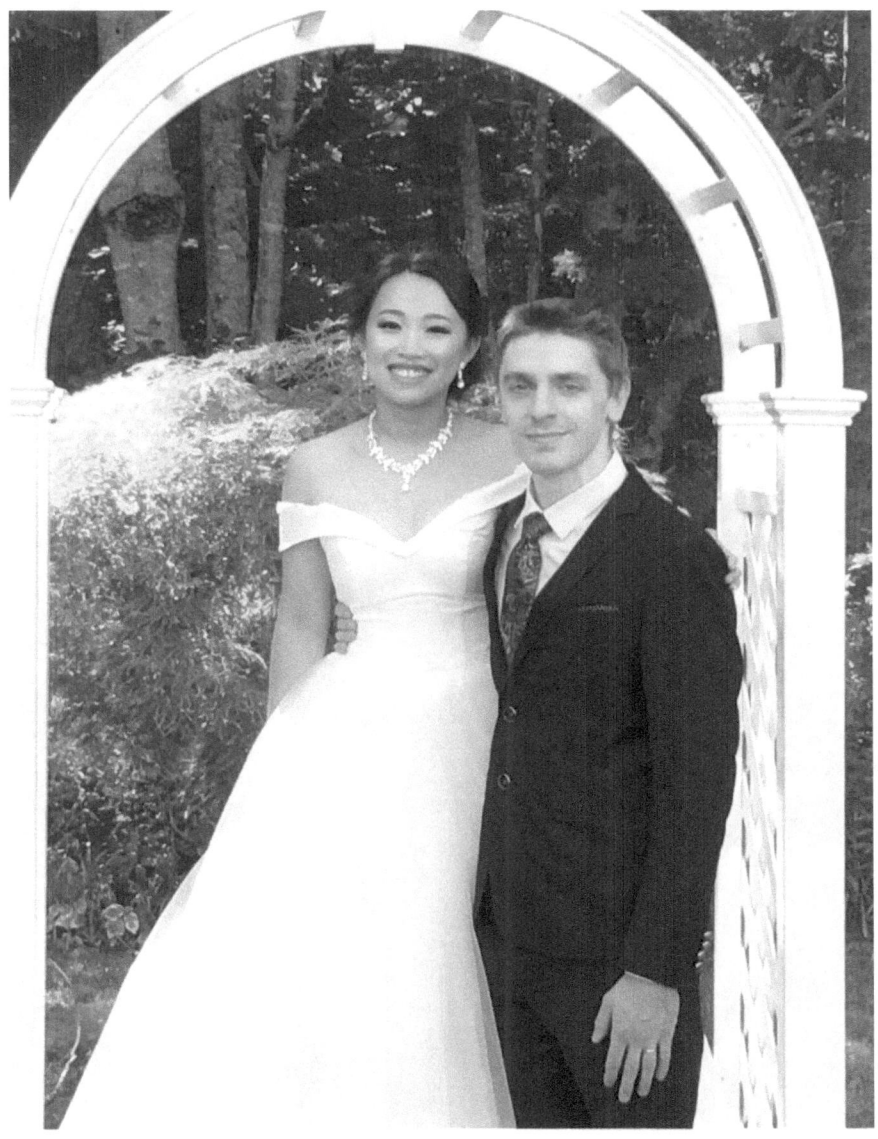

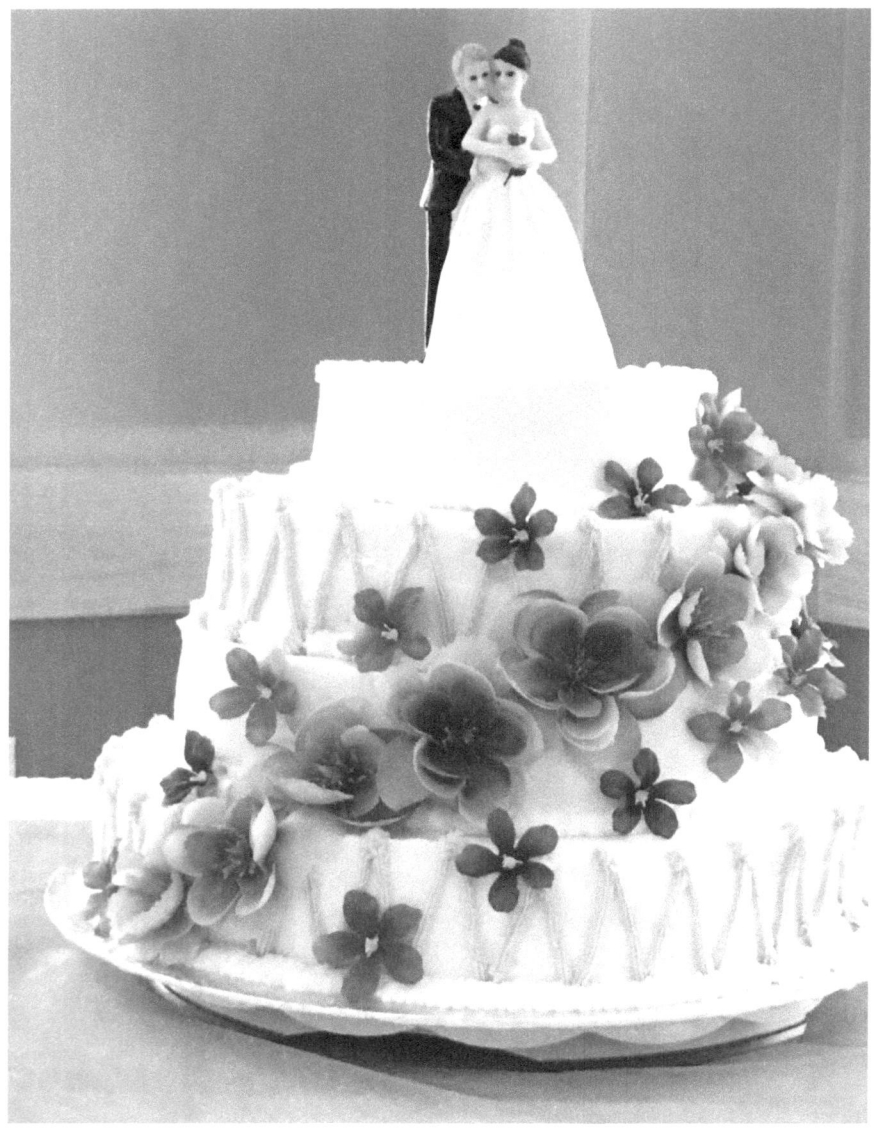

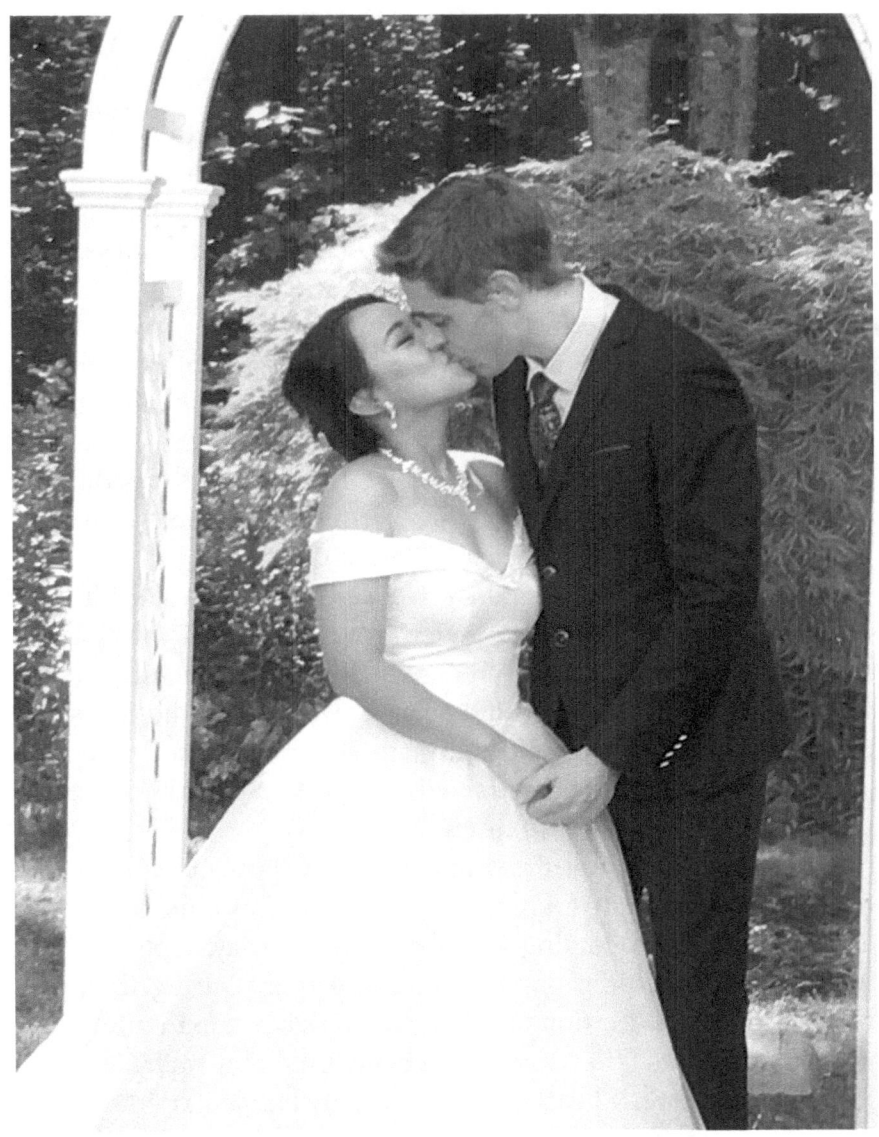

A few days later, I shared my news with James and Bella, as well as the rest of my family. I, of course, told people not to worry because we did not have any official news at that point.

August 13th was my next appointment, an ultrasound. The technologist moved the wand around my right breast for a while then said she needed to leave. She was gone for a while, and when she returned, she had a radiologist with her. I thought to myself, *this can't be good*.

The radiologist informed me that I would need to have a needle biopsy. I was asked for my permission to book the biopsy, or they could follow the protocol, which was to send their request to my family doctor, then he would book the biopsy for me. I was told by the radiologist that giving my permission would expedite the booking for the biopsy. I granted my permission to book the biopsy. The biopsy was booked for August 27th, 2018.

I arrived at Valley Regional Hospital on August 27th. The radiologist was caring, kind, and warm. He warned me that the needle punctures were going to hurt. Before each puncture, he said to me, "I'm sorry," then he would poke me with the needle. The sharp end of the needle plunged into my breast, which caused pain both when it was inserted and retracted. The needle would be plunged into my breast a total of five times.

I went home to await the results from my family physician. The end of August was busy for me as I was preparing my office, resources, and supplies for the coming school year. Wednesday, September 5th was an in-service/prep day for all school staff. During the lunch break, I made the decision to call my doctor's office to inquire about my biopsy results. The secretary informed me that my results had just arrived. I felt my heart begin to race; my hands started shaking. The secretary told me my doctor was open that evening for drop-in appointments, or I could make an appointment for Thursday or Friday. I knew I needed the results sooner than later, so I told her I would come in later that day.

I immediately called my husband and asked him to call the doctor's office back and book a time for me, as I did not want to have to sit and wait.

I was in "panic mode." I stopped to inform my friend, Shelagh, I would be leaving so I could get my results. I went downstairs to the computer lab and gathered my belongings and saw our principal, Maria. I informed her that I needed to leave early. Maria placed her hands on my shoulders and said, "You are going to be okay. You are strong and we are all here for you", as I stood there with tears running down my face.

My brother, Mark, fortunately was home visiting from Alberta, and I called him to find out if he could come with Kevin and me to the doctor's appointment. I drove to my dad's house in Greenwood and picked him up.

The drive to the doctor's office takes ninety minutes, and that day it felt like we were never going to get there. The three of us walked into the waiting room, and I waited for my name to be called. Then I heard a woman's voice say, "Kim Nelson." Kevin and I stood up and walked into the doctor's office.

Dr. Siva entered the room and said, "Hello, Kevin and Kim," and sat down.

I went into a trance-like state after that. I heard the words "The results are not good," then I recall staring straight ahead, the conversation seeming muffled and far away. I heard Kevin say, "It's not in the lymph nodes, right?"

Dr. Siva, in the most kind, caring, gentle manner informed us that the lump was cancer without saying the word cancer. I remember sitting there, slowly processing the words the doctor was saying and thinking to myself, *Oh, oh, oh,* and then it hit me. *He is telling me I have breast cancer.* Tears streamed down my face. I did not utter a word during the conversation.

When I stood up, Dr. Siva approached me and said, "You're going to be okay; you're going to get through this."

I walked through the waiting room, glanced over at my brother, and waved for him to come to the car.

I opened the back passenger side car door, buckled over in a fetal position with my arms wrapped around my waist and began to wail. My head dropped to the seat, and I cried an agonizing cry. Then I realized I had totally lost control in front of Mark and Kevin and tried to pull myself together. I said, "I'm okay. I've had a lot of pent-up emotions over the past two months, and they are all coming out now."

We drove home. I stared out the window. Trees, cars, and people went by as a blur. Kevin and Mark talked, and I sat quietly trying to process the news I had just been given.

After we arrived home, Kevin and Mark informed our family about my cancer diagnosis. Our son and daughter-in-law, James and Bella, had returned to China, so I knew we had to wait to inform them in the morning. Kevin, Mark, and I sat around that Wednesday evening and talked. I was so grateful Mark was with us. He had driven, allowing Kevin to be a passenger on the way home from the doctor's office. I hope Kevin was able to breathe while Mark drove us home.

Mark spoke to our mom, dad, his wife, and his daughter. Kevin told his mom, dad, sister, brother-in-law, and our niece. It was my responsibility to inform my work family. I thought carefully about how to share my news, then crafted the following email:

———————————————

September 5

My doctor is so caring. He delivered my bad news
as gently as possible. I have breast cancer. Next step
is to see the surgeon. For now, I wait. I need to be
home tomorrow; it was a lot to process. Thank you
for your kindness through all this. Your support
means so much to me.

See you Friday.

Kim

I knew I worked with amazing people, and I would have their support. Here are their heartwarming responses to me:

Kim, I am so sorry to hear this. I was hoping for different news but at least now you know and can begin the journey of recovery. Know that we are here to support you in any way you need. Also, when you have put some thought into it, let us know if and what you want us to share with staff. We will get a sub for you tomorrow (and Friday if you think you will need that day too).

Take care and think as many positive thoughts as you can.

M

So sorry to hear. Now you kick the shit out of it!!!

We will be here for you and support you in whatever we can do to help you. I will look after Aesop.

Take care and see you soon.

Cathy

Oh Kim. Please don't worry about anything on our end. I am sorry and you are in all my prayers. Please take good care and know that we are all thinking of you. Jill Gidney

---

Hi Kim,

I am so sorry to hear this. I can assure you that Jill and I will keep this confidential. You know that you are a strong person, and that I will be sending you positive thoughts and prayers. Stay strong and don't

be afraid to pick up the phone for a chat if you need
to hear a friendly voice.

Take care,

Isaac

Maria, PRMS Principal, and Isaac, SMES Principal, sent out an email
to let the staff at both schools know I would be absent; here are the
lovely words they sent out to my fellow colleagues:

> Folks, I just got off the phone with Kim Nelson and
> she received news this afternoon that she will need
> to undergo surgery in the coming weeks for breast
> cancer. This is difficult news for Kim, but she is
> handling the situation amazingly well and is feeling
> positive about the steps ahead. Kim won't be in
> school tomorrow but does plan to be here on Friday.
>
> IMPORTANT: Kim has not had a chance to reach
> her son in China to share the news with him, so
> please don't make any contact with Kim about this
> via social media. Kim said she is ok receiving emails
> but no contact through social media (not even to say
> "thinking of you" or "stay strong" etc.).
>
> Kim is remarkably strong and said she is a great
> example of resilience!

Thursday, September 6th was the first day of school for students and
I would miss that day. I believe it was the first time I ever missed the
first day of school.

That day, I informed James and Bella that I had breast cancer. My
brain was stuck on being positive, so I tried to provide reassurance
that I was fine, and I was going to be fine. James and Bella were so
far away, and I didn't want them to worry about me. In retrospect,
my positive attitude probably did not lessen the blow or the stress of
my news.

On Friday, September 7th, I awoke early, had a shower, ate breakfast, got dressed, then headed to work. I opened the car door, sat down, started the car, and held onto the steering wheel. I took several deep breaths, put the car in drive, and listened to the wheels scrunch down on the gravel in the driveway. I turned left and could feel my heart pounding while I continued to take deep breaths. I was worried I may fall apart once I saw my colleagues. How on earth was I going to walk in the school like everything in my world was the same as the last time I saw them?

To my surprise, when I entered, I was greeted with smiles and casual conversation. I felt so at ease that I went about my morning routine and let go of "how was cancer going to change my life?" All my colleagues were so respectful and asked if it was permissible to give me a hug and, of course, I said, "Yes." My boundaries were clear to me; I could not talk about my diagnosis, but I could be "me" at work. I felt so relieved once I got through day one.

All my colleagues at the elementary school were also so respectful the following week. I learned quickly that I was going to be able to function and do my job until I received further information from my doctor. I rounded out Friday with dear friends coming to visit me, along with my brother. We had lots of fun and loads of laughs.

Kindness, care, and support followed in September when I encountered the difficult days.

September 11

Hey Maria,

I am struggling today and need to stay home tonight. I have put on my brave face all day; however, I am exhausted and just want to go home and try and get some sleep. I will stay for the staff meeting.

Kim

September 11

Maria and Cathy,

I appreciate your support more than I can express adequately. I needed to be home tonight to deal with my anxiety; I cannot even begin to explain how immeasurable it is for me.

I am so scared about my appointment tomorrow, which I didn't realize until I got home tonight. I will be coming to school tomorrow; if I am late, please forgive me. I have decided to take a sedative to help me sleep. Thank you, thank you, thank you,

See you in the morning,

Kim

September 11

We are always here to support you. Sending you lots of love and will see you in the morning.

Cathy

September 11

Kim, hope you are sleeping now. When you check email tomorrow remember you will get through this. There is a positive to your situation already (clear lymph nodes) and every hour puts you closer to recovery and good health.

See you tomorrow,

Maria

September 12

Thank you, Maria. Your kind words inspire me to
keep the faith and stay positive. I am just anxious
about the appointment today.

Thanks!!!!

Love, Kim

On September 12th, Kevin and I visited the surgeon, who provided details about my test results. I sat on the end of the table while he felt the lump and talked about the options for surgery. I could hear words coming from his mouth, but I did not understand anything he was talking about. I had no idea how intense my stress level was and, in my effort, to cope with the stress, I blocked the information by zoning out. My only thought was, *Take the breast so I can live my life.*

When we left, I remembered certain words and phrases the doctor had used, but I did not have the information in the proper context. I thought I had the option of a lumpectomy and perhaps my cancer fit into the "in situ" category, which meant the cancer cells were lumped together and had not spread. Kevin later informed me that the doctor had said I had aggressive breast cancer. My official diagnosis, I later learned, was invasive ductal carcinoma with accompanying high-grade ductal carcinoma.

It was important to me to inform my administrators immediately. I sent out the following email and their responses came steadfastly:

September 12

Hey gals,

Dr. Clark provided great information to us. I will
be having a mastectomy on October 18. Thank you
so much for all your support as I navigate through
this journey.

See you in the morning.

Love,

Kim

September 12

Glad the conversation with the doctor was helpful. If you need anything between now and October 18, or after the surgery, just let me know. You can do this!!!

Maria

Hi Kim,

Glad to hear they can get you in right away, and that you got all the information you needed. We can chat tomorrow as I know how tired and draining this must be.

Lots of love,

Cathy

Hi Kim,

Great to hear from you. No worries on tomorrow night :) I am sure we can make it work. Maybe tomorrow we can chat a little bit if you have a minute to spare :)

Isaac

On September 26th, we visited the doctor again, and he outlined option one: remove the breast, or option two: if the cancer had spread toward the axilla, armpit, then lymph nodes would be removed along with the breast and sent to pathology. The surgeon had a consent form for me to sign. I was feeling numb and with my shaky right hand, I signed the form while tears trickled down my face. The surgeon asked us if we would like some privacy, and I said, "No, it's just disconcerting to sign a form to remove a body part."

Once I returned home, I sent an email to my administrators to inform them about my next steps, and again I was uplifted by their care and compassion.

September 26

After our discussion with the surgeon, it is apparent that I need to have the right breast removed. Apparently, the cancer is invasive, which means there are other distorted cells and they do not know if they are benign, so I don't want to take any chances.

October 18 is still the surgery date. See you in the morning. Isaac and Jill, see you Tuesday.

Kim

Thanks for the update, Kim.

Better to get it all now. Thinking of you and let me know if there is anything I can do for you.

Cathy

Hi Kim,

Sorry to hear this. Please know I am thinking of you and hoping for only positive things :)

Isaac

September 26

I want to let you know today was incredibly difficult as I had held out hope for a partial mastectomy. Some of the info given at our first consult, I did not compute. Learning that there are other areas of concern hit me harder than I expected. I will be at work tomorrow. I needed to take something to help me sleep. I don't plan to be late. If I am, please bear with me.

Kim

Kim, I am so sorry to hear that you have received more difficult news. We are thinking about you and want to support in any way that we can. I'm not at school tomorrow, and if you feel that school is a good place for you to be tomorrow, I am happy to support that. We do understand if you need us to book a sub to though. Sometimes keeping busy is the best thing you can do. Having said this, tomorrow morning will be the whole school assembly where we will be drawing for some prizes and then showing a video about Terry Fox. Perhaps you might find it easier to be working in your office during the later part of this assembly when we are showing that video. I'll leave that to your judgement. We do have you slotted in to do one of the crossing points during the walk/run, so please see Cathy if that is not something you feel you can do. If you can't do it, we need to get someone else as we don't have "extra people" right now. Being out in the fresh air and cheering on the kids as they walk by might be great for you though.

Take care and think positive!

M

September 27

Hi Maria

Thanks for your kindness and support. The visit with the surgeon hit me hard. I was so exhausted this morning I contacted Cathy to get a sub. I went back to bed and did not wake up until noon. I knew I was tired, so it was a good decision to be home today.

My plan is to see you tomorrow. Again, thank you for your support; I appreciate more than words can say.

Kim

September 28

Hey gals,

I have a note that I would like you to share with staff.

Thanks,

Kim

To keep my colleagues informed at both schools, I sent out an update. This is my first note to staff:

A Note from Kim–September 28, 2018

Dear PRMS/SMES staff,

I want to give you all an update about the next steps for me. I visited the surgeon for a second time this past week. I had held out hope that I might have the option of a partial mastectomy. The doctor reviewed my tests and disclosed that I have other "distorted" cells near the cancer cells, which could be problematic later. Learning this news, I have made the decision to have a full mastectomy (removal of right breast).

The surgery will take place in Kentville on October 18; I need to be there early (6:30 am) so that preliminary tests can be completed before the surgery at 1:00 that afternoon. The doctor tells me that I should only be in the hospital one night and go home on Friday, October 19th.

Recovery time will last four to six weeks.

When the breast is removed, samples will be taken from my lymph nodes (this is a standard procedure). Once the pathology is back from the lymph node samples, I will find out whether I need chemotherapy, radiation, both or none. The amount of time I will be away is uncertain at this point as everything will depend on the lymph node testing.

I am doing fairly well; this past week has been challenging to say the least. Having a doctor read the consent form to remove a body part was unsettling and frightening. It is difficult to explain my emotions as they are so foreign to me. I shall keep my positive attitude through the fear and angst because I know I have lots of "outrageous love" supporting me through this time.

Thank you for your hugs, conversations, nods, winks, kindness, positivity, and support. There are no words to express how grateful I am to have you in my life.

Love,

Kim

SURGERY AND NEXT STEPS

I worked until Wednesday, October 17th with the uncertainty of my return. I had imagined I would need radiation after my surgery and would return to work in a few months. I felt it was best to inform students I would be away, and I did not want to share my diagnosis with any of the students. The students I work with are dealing with their own issues, so I did not want anyone worrying about me. I prepared a note for teachers to read to the students. It was important for me to let the kids know I would be leaving for a while and that a new counsellor would be there for all of them. I sent the following email to my administrator along with the attached announcement.

ANNOUNCEMENT

For: October 15, 2018 –To be read during SSR on Monday

I would like to share some information with you from Mrs. Nelson.

Mrs. Nelson is having surgery, which will take place this Thursday, October 18th. Wednesday, October 17th will be her last day with us for a while. Mrs. Nelson is uncertain about her return date. Once the doctor has given his permission, she will be back to hang out with us. Surgery is personal and private, so I do not have any other information to share with you now. Mr. Higgins will be in for Mrs. Nelson

while she is away. Let's make sure we make him
feel welcome.

I then reached out to the Cancer Care Patient Navigator to ask for
support. Below is the response I received from her:

Thank you, Kim, for reaching out before your
surgery! You are certainly in good hands with
Dr. Clark.

In case the nursing staff forget to give you:

- ensure you ask for a soft form (great if you
  are headed out to town and just want a more
  uniform look until you can be properly fitted for
  a prosthesis, if you want one)

- the heart-shape pillow and drain bag—a great
  comfort for the discomfort under the arm area.

- The breast exercise booklet—some you start
  on the very next day, others not until the drain
  is removed.

I would love to connect with you post op—would it
be ok if I called your home early next week?? Or you
can certainly call me, the number will be below for
my office. Look forward to talking with you.

Call for any questions!

Dianna Hutt

It was important for me to say goodbye to my elementary school
family as I would be finished on Tuesday, October 16th, so I wanted
to go there that morning. Leaving the school on Wednesday, October
17th was difficult as I had no sense of what lay ahead the next day or
in the days that followed the surgery.

Below is my update for October, which sums up what transpired.

My October update to staffs

October 18th began at 5:00 a.m., arriving at the hospital at 6:30 a.m. I slipped into my johnny shirt and waited patiently. At 9:00 a.m., I was wheeled to nuclear medicine to have a dye procedure. The dye procedure consisted of four needles poked into my nipple with no freezing—OUCH! I then had pictures completed two hours later. Kevin and I again sat and waited; we were told the surgery would take place at 1:30. There were medical emergencies that morning, so my surgery was delayed. Kevin and I walked to the OR at 3:00, and I walked into the operating room at approximately 3:35. I hugged Kevin, and he gently kissed my right breast and said, "Bye." We hugged tightly once more then I walked to the room. The room was big; bright lights shone on the table and several people were present. The anesthesiologist introduced himself then placed a mask on my face; this is my last conscious memory. When I awoke, I recall crying and the nurse quietly and calmly telling me I was in recovery, and I was doing well. My next memory is being wheeled to my hospital room.

Kevin expected the surgery to last an hour and a half; unfortunately, the surgery took three hours. The surgeon had to remove lymph nodes he felt could be problematic. I was taken to a room by 8:30 p.m. and was able to enjoy an orange popsicle. It tasted soooo good! I stayed in the hospital until Saturday. My blood pressure was alarmingly high during and after surgery, so they kept me an additional day. I have two drains—one in my chest and one in my armpit. It is our hope the drains will be removed this week.

My family visited with me, and when Kevin and I were alone he shared sweet, caring, supportive messages, which had been sent to us from our friends. I want you to know how much we appreciate all the love, support, and kindness you have shown us. It has provided us with so much comfort.

I am doing my exercises four times a day and will begin additional stretches this coming weekend. I am resting comfortably, and Kevin has been taking excellent care of me.

I know I have said thank you often. Please know your hugs, talks, and well wishes helped me get through one of the most difficult days I have ever experienced. I miss all of you, and I can't wait until we are walking the halls together again.

Much love,

Kim & Kevin (and Bear, Koko, and Luna)

I received the following heartwarming messages after my first update:

October 22

Such a warm and compassionate update. No surprise coming from you. You are a strong individual and will make it through this! Let us know if you need anything at all. I will forward to staff later tonight. People will likely ask if you are up for visitors. How would you like us to respond to this?

Take care,

Maria

Hi Maria, I have lots of family around this week and I do not have my doctor appointments scheduled yet. Perhaps people could check in with me next week.

Love, Kim

October 23

Update from Kim.….Also, Kim indicated to me that she has lots of family around this week so if folks are considering a visit, next week would likely be better timing. Please check with her before you decide to drop by.

Maria

After my surgery, I focused on rest, completing my exercises four times a day, eating well, and going out for walks. I was anxious and hopeful about my pathology results. The surgeon expected the results to take three to four weeks.

I received a phone call from the doctor's office, and I was scheduled for an appointment on November 6th, 2018. The results were not as I had hoped, so once again I zoned out and Kevin listened. Dr. Clark informed me that I was going to need chemotherapy and radiation treatments.

When we returned to the truck, Kevin had tears running down his cheeks. I said, "It's going to be ok. I know it is scary, but we'll get through this." In a comforting voice, I told him, "I am not the first person to receive chemotherapy, and I won't be the last."

I sent a message to my administrators to give them an update:

November 6

Hey gals,

I received my pathology results tonight and they were not as good as I had hoped they would be. Lymph nodes were removed during surgery and some of my lymph nodes are cancerous. What that now means is I will need chemo and radiation. The chemo and radiation will not be scheduled until I have recovered for six weeks, which puts us in early

December. I will type an email tomorrow, which you can share with staff to give them an update.

Love,

Kim

Hi Kim,

I have thought about you all day. I am sure the news was not what you were hoping for. Your positive energy will carry into the next stage. You are on my mind and giving you big hugs.

Love you,

Cathy

I'm sorry to hear this news. Keep in mind it only means that your path to recovery will just be a bit longer with more steps. Keep thinking positively and do what ever you need to do to get healthy.

Let us know if you need anything in the coming days and weeks.

We miss you at school.

M

Hi Kim,

I am seeing this now as I was out with meetings and coaching last night. I am so sorry to hear that news. I am sending you positive thoughts and prayers. I know you can do this!

Hang in there and keep staying strong. I would like to stop by for a quick visit sometime if you would be okay with that. Please let me know.

Take care,

Isaac

I spent the remainder of November processing my next steps and feeling uneasy about chemotherapy. I was diligent with my arm exercises and went out for walks regularly. I sent out an update for November.

_____

November 7, 2018

Hello dear friends,

Thursday, November 8th will mark three weeks into my recovery from surgery. I am doing great so far. Each day I feel stronger. I am doing my exercises three times per day with the goal of gaining full mobility in my right arm. Physically, I feel well, I am sleeping well, and I am eating well.

Yesterday, Kevin and I visited Dr. Clark to receive my pathology report. I showered, put on my make-up, and dressed in "real clothes" (not my sweats as in previous visits) for I was feeling so positive. The conversation began with "Parts of your report are worrisome . . ." I then sat up straight and proceeded to listen carefully to the worrisome components. To summarize the important parts: I had 26 lymph nodes removed during the surgery and some of the lymph nodes are cancerous. What this means is I will need to have both chemo and radiation treatments. These treatments will not begin until I have six weeks of recovery time completed (tomorrow will be three weeks). Dr. Clark said on average there will probably be six rounds of chemo and three radiation treatments.

My hope for this visit was to hear that the lymph nodes were clear, and I would need radiation, so this news was unsettling. I am now allowing the information to sink in and gain my next batch of strength to get through the next part of this journey. A positive aspect, though, is I should be able to have my chemo treatments in Kentville—for this, I am most appreciative.

Prayers, positivity, faith, love, hope, support, and strength are welcome to be sent my way. I am feeling fearful once again, however, I know I have an army of family and friends cheering me on!

Love to you all and I miss you dearly,

Kim

DECEMBER

In December, I continued to do my exercises and practice breathing activities, as I was getting nervous about my first chemotherapy treatment. I had several kind, thoughtful messages during the month, which I am sharing with you below. There are no words to adequately express how comforting these messages were, how much each person checking in with me did to fill my heart and soul with strength. The uncertainty of what was to come often swirled in my thoughts, and I did my best to push away my fears.

December 2

Hi Maria,

Giving gifts is an art. Those who give the gift give great thought to the person receiving the gift. You, my Pine Ridge family, warmed my heart with a homemade advent tree. The time, energy, and effort you put into this gift for me warms my heart. I truly am excited about uncovering each numbered gift.

You all have a special place in my heart. I am truly blessed to have you all in my life and right now in my corner.

I have the house all decorated so if you need a snowman fix, come on over. You all have a standing invitation. Again, thank you for touching my heart. A couple of pics to share with you.

Love

Kim

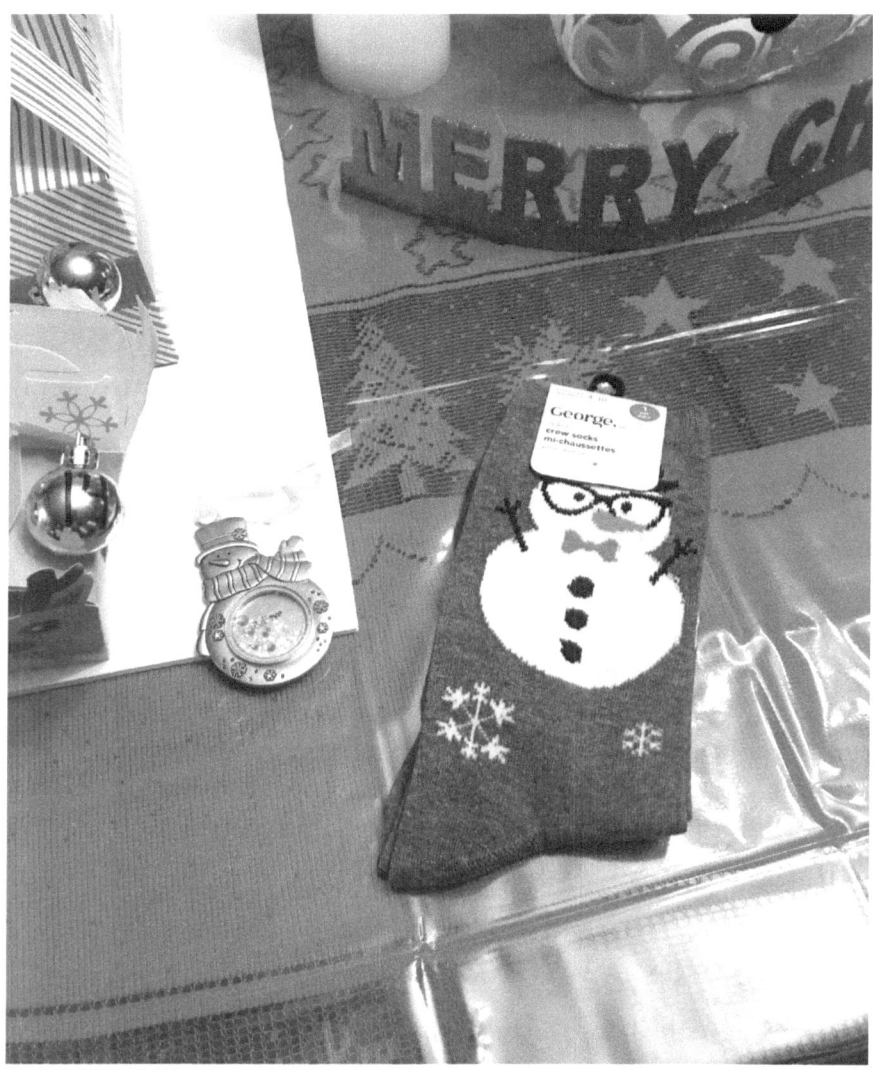

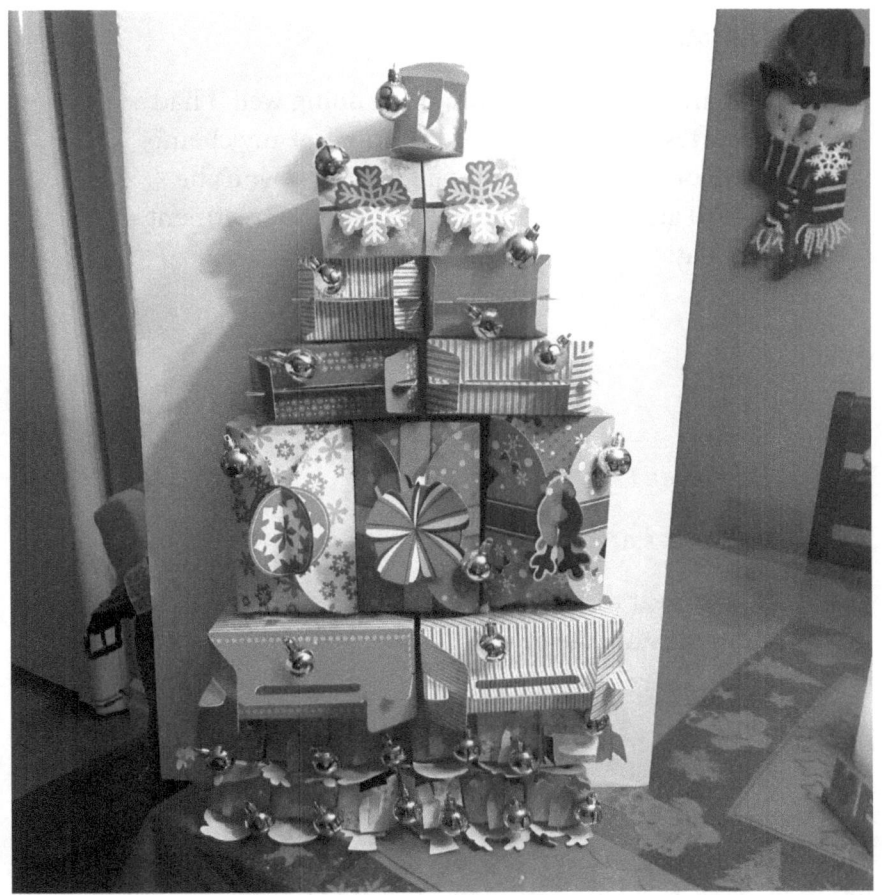

December 3

I missed seeing you last week, but I hear that you are doing fantastic. Hope the holiday season has you feeling strong, positive, and loved!

If you feel up to it, drop by on December 13th for the school-wide turkey dinner!

M

Hey Maria

It is nice to hear from you. I am doing well. I had a few tests last week in preparation for my chemo. I will be thinking of you on the 13th. I won't be able to attend; it will be my first chemo treatment that day.

Love,

Kim

December 12

Hello Maria,

It was great to see you today. Could you please pass along this update to staff.

Thanks,

Kim

In December I also met my oncologist, Dr. Merryweather, who provided a thorough overview of the chemotherapy and follow-up between chemo treatments. My December overview outlines my next steps in this journey.

Hello folks,

I wanted to give you one last update before you begin your Christmas break. I dropped into the school today and had fun hanging out with the Core Team during their meeting today. My heart is filled with joy each time I come in for a visit. I appreciate the hugs and encouraging words.

Physically I am feeling great. I am going out for walks and doing my exercises. Phase two of my

exercise program is proving to be a little more
challenging. I visited a physiotherapist last week
to ensure I had not hurt myself from the exercises;
I had been experiencing quite a bit of pain in my
right bicep. The muscle is "tight", so I need to
persevere, go slow, and keep pushing until I am
"comfortably uncomfortable."

I have undergone several tests in preparation
for my chemo treatments. I had a MUGA, a.k.a.
heart function test, an ultrasound, and a bone
scan. Chantel—this info is just for you: during the
ultrasound, I had the dye test, which causes a flush
of heat throughout your body and the sensation
of wetting your pants. I will begin my treatments
tomorrow, December 13th at 8:15 a.m.; I am
thankful that my treatments will take place at the
Kentville hospital. Although the oncologist told me
the chemo will take four hours to administer, Kevin
(my hubby) and I will be there longer as they cannot
create my chemo-cocktail until, as they put it, my
bum is in the chair. The schedule for my chemo
will be every third Thursday for six rounds, which
will have me completing this part of the journey
in March.

I will need three sessions of radiation that will
take place in Halifax. I have not yet met with a
radiologist. Radiation can not occur until the chemo
treatments have been completed. I hope these
treatments will occur in April.

I want to wish all of you a very Merry Christmas. I
hope your holidays are filled with laughter and love.
It is the time of year to make memories with our

family and friends. I miss you all dearly and look forward to seeing you again soon!

Much love,

Kim

My friend Shelagh C checked in on me often and I want her to know how incredibly grateful I am for her support throughout my journey. In December, Shelagh sent me the following message:

December 8

Hey there,

Well, second storm day in a row and I'm not gonna lie . . . it's been great! I got some schoolwork done but I also finished knitting a pair of socks for my son's girlfriend and did a bit of tidying and organizing in the house. I managed to get my parcels sent off to my dad and brothers in Ontario, which I've been slow getting done.

One of my favourite things over the past few days has been listening to the CBC! I rarely get to listen during weekdays and it's such a treat—the programs are very different from the ones on the weekend. Weekday listening reminds me of being on holidays because that is the only time I get to do that!

I am hoping that the days since your chemo have been manageable. From friends I have spoken with, it seems like it affects each person differently. I am imagining you all snuggled up in your "nest" on the couch, surrounded by your puppies and all those beautiful Christmas lights. Such a lovely place to heal.

Sending big hugs your way. Talk soon.

Shelagh

My response to Shelagh's message:

———————————————

December 19

Hi Shelagh, it is always so great to hear from you. I love your updates and the photo you sent me. They truly lift my spirits. Last week was the most challenging to date. I was hit with angst and fear when I went for chemo.

I was a little nauseous Thursday night, which freaked me out a little. I had a weepy Friday, then Saturday morning my mom called and told me my cousin had died. My cousin, Patti, has been battling bone and blood cancer for the past three-and-a-half years. That news hit me hard. I have felt like a nervous wreck.

I am feeling a little better with each day that passes. I have been thinking about Patti so much I cannot seem to settle during the day or night. The funeral service is tomorrow, but I am not going to attend. I am not strong enough physically or emotionally right now.

I have been reciting the mantra you said your yoga teacher uses: calm mind, calm breath, calm body.

My brother, Mark, has been awesome. He calls me twice a week; I do not know what we talk about for almost an hour—but we manage to talk.

I bet you thoroughly enjoyed having the past two days off. What a great break for you to have. Only two-and-a-half more days and you get some well-deserved down time.

Shelagh, I am so grateful for you checking on me. I am so lucky to have such an amazing friend.

I want to wish you and your family a very Merry Christmas and I look forward to walking the halls with you in 2019. May you make wonderful, family memories this Christmas.

Take good care and relax.

Love, Kim

CHEMO BEGINS

My first chemotherapy treatment occurred on Thursday, December 13th. I had been informed that I would receive the chemo cocktail of FEC-D. Kevin and I arrived at 8:30 a.m. I am at a loss to find words to express how I was feeling that morning. We were called in and were told to choose a chair. Kevin and I chose a spot in the corner, which also had lots of windows. The nurse came over and explained the process I would go through. My chemo drugs were ordered through the pharmacy located in the hospital.

An IV was placed in my arm. The first liquid through the IV was to flush my vein, and when the chemo drugs arrived, I would receive three different drugs: 5-fluorouracil, epirubicin and cyclophosphamide (this is the FEC part of the drugs). The epirubicin, bright red, was housed in two large syringes. The nurse connected the syringe to my IV line and gently and slowly began to push the drug through my IV. Once the two syringes were completed, I was then hooked up with a drip for the next two drugs. The first day was long and tiring. We did not leave until later in the afternoon. When I arrived home, my stomach felt upset, and I began to feel panicky. After deep breaths and using the washroom, I felt better and decided to lie down and rest.

During my first visit, I met Dianna Hutt, Cancer Patient Navigator, who introduced herself to me and gave me a gift bag. While Dianna and I were talking, she noticed my right hand and arm looked swollen. Dianna said it looked like lymphedema. Dianna recommended I contact Julie Skaling who specializes in lymphatic drainage massage. I remember I had read something about the possibility of lymphedema occurring after a mastectomy. Since I was not interested in learning more about it, I did not know this was going to become a life-time issue for me. Since twenty-six lymph nodes had been removed, my lymphatic system was now compromised, and I had to re-route the lymphatic fluid through exercises, which I learned from Julie.

I also learned I needed to take needles between chemo treatments. Each chemo treatment, I was instructed I may need between seven to ten needles. The medication was to help increase my white blood cell count. I was given the option of having health care come to my home to give me the needle, but I felt I could give myself the needle independently. I recall standing in the bathroom when I administered the first needle thinking to myself, *I don't know if I can do this*. I pinched my stomach area, pushed the needle in my skin, pushed the medication in, then pulled it out. Whew, I did it!! I soon became a whiz giving myself injections.

I spent December decorating the house for the holidays, wrapping presents, and feeling thankful for our family and friends. Our family gathered for our traditional Christmas day breakfast. Our table was surrounded by James, Bella (our son and daughter-in-law), my mom and dad, Ron and Gloria, Kevin's mom and dad, Ruth and Gordon, as well as Kelly, Brent, and Alxys (my sister-in law, brother-in-law, and our niece) and of course Kevin and me. We enjoyed ham, hash browns, toast, eggs, coffee, tea, and juice. After breakfast, some of opened our gifts. While at our house, James, Bella, Kevin and I would open the gifts we all gave to one another. We then relocated to Kelly and Brent's house to watch them open the gifts they gave to each other. The finale of our day ends at Ruth and Gordon's house to enjoy Christmas dinner and then we open our gifts from them. We have a full day of family, which results in laughs, a few tears (from some of the gifts that were given), and much love.

I decided at the end of the month to have my head shaved. My hair was beginning to fall out in my hand, so I thought it best to take it off. It was very strange to see my bald reflection in the hair salon. The reality of my diagnosis was staring me in the face.

Kevin and I rang in the new year at home watching the countdown on television.

HAPPY NEW YEAR

My second chemo appointment occurred on Thursday, January 3rd, 2019. I did well during my treatment and had my loving husband, Kevin, by my side. Kevin and I met some incredible people during my treatments. I spent the month focusing on arm exercises, bundling up and going for walks, and healthy eating habits.

My third chemo appointment was scheduled on Thursday, January 24th. A new nurse assisted me this time. For some reason, I had a knot in my stomach. I was worried about the placement of my intravenous needle, which was located on the top of my left hand. I cannot explain why I felt so uneasy. Perhaps my body knew something was going to go wrong that day.

As the nurse began to push the epirubicin drug in my IV, she appeared to be struggling. Then she asked me if I felt any burning or pain, and I said no. But when I looked at my arm, where the IV was located, I noticed my skin protruding, and I knew that was not normal.

Next thing I knew, the nurse left, the oncologist came over to the chair I was sitting in to receive my treatment, looked at my arm and said she was going to make some phone calls. Kevin and I we were left sitting in the oncology department for a few hours. At one point, I asked the nurse if I was going to receive the rest of my treatments and she said, "No." Kevin and I passed the time talking or playing on our phones. I was disappointed that my treatment was cancelled. What I came to learn was the drug did not go through the IV, instead it went under my skin. Dr. Merryweather informed us she was going to investigate best practices for the epirubicin leak in my arm.

A few hours later, the pharmacist arrived with medication, and I was given instructions. I would rotate the application of the medication, which needed to be done for a twenty-four-hour period. This meant I would need to apply the drug and ensure I set my alarm every two hours through the night to put the medication on my arm.

I was so exhausted after those twenty-four hours. One of the drugs had a strong, unpleasant smell. I tried to ensure my arm did not touch the blankets.

Since my treatment had been cancelled, it was rescheduled for Thursday, January 31st.

January 13, 2019

Hello folks,

I hope you all celebrated the holidays with family and friends and have many cherished memories from your time together. I truly do want to say thank you again for the advent tree you gave me; it truly was the best gift ever. Every morning, I woke up and felt excited to find the box I would open. Thank you for your generosity, I truly appreciate you thinking of me.

I have had two chemo treatments and so far, I am handling the medicine well. The second treatment, I felt a fatigue I have never experienced before. Once it hits, I need to sleep; there is no fighting it, one must give in and rest. I have developed lymphedema in my right arm. This is due to the lymph nodes that were removed during my surgery. Lymph nodes normally drain in the armpit, neck, and groin. Some of my lymph nodes do not have a path so fluid is accumulating in my right arm and hand. I am now seeing a physiotherapist on a weekly basis for gentle massage with the purpose of re-routing the fluid and protein to a new location.

I will be staying close to home for the next couple of months as my immune system is compromised with the chemo treatments. I have become quite proficient in giving myself a needle post-chemo. Since the chemo depletes my white blood cells, I need to give myself a needle anywhere from seven to ten times to help build up the white blood cells. My poor left arm has become a human pin cushion as I need to go for bloodwork three to four times between treatments. My final treatment will be March 28th, then I will need to wait a few weeks before I go for radiation. I have not yet connected with a radiologist at this point.

I am hoping that I can get out for daily walks again soon; the weather and my energy level have kept me in the house more than I would like at this point. I am grateful for my dogs, for they keep me entertained during the day and give lots of great cuddles daily. All in all, I am feeling quite well. My appetite is good, I am sleeping fairly well, and I am trying to do little things around the house when I can so I can get up and move around as often as I can.

I miss you all dearly and I miss hanging out with the students. I hope you are all doing well. I look forward to seeing your beautiful faces in the next few months and will openly welcome bear hugs from all.

Love,

Kim

January 31st marked my third chemotherapy treatment. I had no issues during this treatment and felt relieved that the first three sessions were complete.

February 2019

Hello folks,

I was so happy to see so many of you on Friday when I was in the building. For those of you I missed, I will look forward to seeing you the next time I'm able to get back for a visit.

I had my third chemo treatment last Thursday, January 31st. My treatment, originally scheduled for January 24th, did not work out. The IV needle moved, or my vein blew so the concern was that some of the chemo meds went under my skin or in my tissue. As a preventative, I had to leave with a topical solution to apply every two hours for a twenty-four-hour period. Then I was on a three-hour schedule applying topical solution and hydrocortisone. I was exhausted by the time I needed my treatment. This treatment marks the halfway point. Yea!! The next three treatments will consist of only one drug; three more to go.

Kevin and I will be celebrating our birthdays this coming weekend; mine is the 9th and Kevin's is the 10th. It will be a low-key weekend; many of our family members have had colds, so they are avoiding me and Kevin for now. I am happy to be marking another year; I really appreciate everything so much more now.

I can not begin to express how elated I was to see many of you on Friday. I appreciated your hugs, kind words, and continued support and love. My heart was so full when I left, I thought I might explode with happiness. I am truly blessed to have you all in my circle of friends.

I hope you have a wonderful February; March break is just around the corner. Until I see you again, take good care of yourselves.

Much love,

Kim

My fourth treatment occurred on February 25th. My white cell count was low, so I needed to wait an additional week to allow my body to recover. The fourth drug I would receive was called docetaxel. My oncologist informed me that this drug would cause dryness, along with other side effects. I recall her telling me that I would either feel as though I'd been hit by a dinky truck or a Mack truck. I was hoping for the dinky truck, but of course that's not what happened.

After my first Docetaxel treatment, I felt well the first two days, then my body just ached. I was tired, sore, and had little energy. These symptoms lasted three or four days, then I felt like myself again. My second Docetaxel treatment occurred on March 18th, 2019. I sent my next update on March 28th, 2019:

Hello ladies,

I wanted to give you an update: I have one more treatment—can I get a "hell yes," which should take place on April 8th. I was informed yesterday that my white count is great, so I have no more needles to give myself. I will have an appointment with Dr. Merryweather next week, then more bloodwork on

Friday, April 5th to ensure all my bloodwork is okay for my final treatment.

I have had to deal with some challenging side effects from this drug Docetaxel. I cannot tell you how glad I will be when the chemo is all over. I have visited with the radiologist and her team; what a wonderful group of ladies. I will need twenty-five rounds of radiation, which means I will need to stay in Halifax for five weeks as the radiation takes place everyday Monday through Friday. I don't have an expected start date right now, but it is supposed to be three to four weeks after my last chemo.

I am hoping the radiation treatments will be completed in early June. It is my hope and intention to return to work either the week of June 10th or June 17th depending on my last treatment. I think it will be beneficial for my mental and physical health to get my "school legs" under me.

As always, I miss you all and cannot wait until we see each other again. Take good care!

Love,

Kim

Kim, it is great to hear that you are coming into the home stretch and soon this will be behind you. We will be happy to have you back whenever you are able to return.

Maria

Thanks for the update, happy to hear you are getting
to the end. I would be so happy to see you whenever
you are ready to come back. June would be an
awesome time to return!!

Hugs,

Cathy

My next update concerns the decision we had to make for our
fur baby.

March 2019

Hello PRMS and SMES staffs:

It is March and I am sure you are counting down the
days until your break, especially with report card
writing. I hope you can enjoy and relax once the
break comes and have all this behind you.

I had chemo treatment number four February25th;
this is the beginning of a new drug being
administered. Docetaxel is a drip drug, which
only takes an hour to give (although we are at the
oncology department for four hours). My left arm
has been pricked and prodded so much; I think it
would like to go on strike. My right hand was used
for the fourth chemo treatment. The side effects
of the Docetaxel have been challenging for me.
Physically I have felt so great, and this drug knocked
me down. I experienced pain all over. It would be
like going to the gym and doing a five-hour workout
when you have not worked out in a long time, then
trying to move the next day. I was so uncomfortable
it was difficult to sleep through the night last
Thursday, Friday, Saturday, and Sunday. Another
side effect is dryness; my lips and mouth have taken

the brunt of this effect. I don't have much of an appetite because my mouth is so dry, I can't really taste anything. I can honestly say this is the first time since my diagnosis I am struggling.

After my chemo treatment, we came home and our oldest dog, Bear, was not in decent shape. Bear could not walk, as his back legs would not work. We called the vet and made the agonizing decision to have him put to sleep. Bear was fourteen years old and brought much joy to our family over the years. The vet and the assistant were so wonderful with us. They put a blanket down for Bear and we sat on the floor with him patting him and talking to him. When he passed, he was lovingly leaning against Kevin, having his ears rubbed. Koko and Luna are coming around this week, and we are trying to adjust to life without our precious Bear.

I have an appointment with a radiologist on Monday, March 11th. Once I meet with the radiologist, I will learn what the treatment steps will be once the chemo is done. I am truly thankful there are only two more chemo treatments to go.

I hope you enjoy your March Break, and it is filled with family, fun, and relaxation. I miss you all and look forward to seeing you soon.

Love,

Kim

The side effects of the Docetaxel lasted a few days, then the pain lessened, and I could get back to my exercises and go out for walks. I learned that my radiologist, Dr. Cwajna, was going to be outlining my radiation treatments. My first appointment was to get tattoos for the radiation treatment. During the month of March, my

Auntie Jeanette died, and I was heartbroken. Kevin and I drove to Amherst on March 10th to attend her visitation, then travelled back to Halifax to stay overnight as the next day I had my appointment with radiology.

On March 11th, I met with Dr. W. Labyslawa Cwajna, radiologist. Dr. Cwajna discussed her recommendations for my radiation treatment. Dr. Cwajna provided details about best practices and recommended I receive twenty-five radiation treatments. I was given a booklet with information about radiation along with a contact person, if I had any questions during the radiation treatment phase.

Before beginning my breast radiation, I met with a wonderful lady, a radiographer, who informed me about the procedure of marking my body with four pinpoint tattoo marks for my radiation treatment. The tattoos are placed in precise locations to direct the radiation during treatment. Every treatment is aimed at the same location to prevent recurrence and spare healthy tissue. Precise measurements of my body were completed so that I would fit snugly on the table when the radiation treatments were to begin. My head was cradled, and my feet were resting comfortably against the adjusted table.

SPRING 2019

April 7th, I received a beautiful gift from my friends at SMES.

THANK YOU

Dear SMES family:

It is with much gratitude I say thank you for the
lovely gifts you delivered to my home. I was so
excited to learn the package on the front veranda
was for me. Kevin often leaves packages for
his plumber friends, so I thought it was either
something he left out or something that had been
dropped off for him. Then he told me the package
was for me.

I appreciate everything you gave to me. It really
warms my heart, more than you will ever know,
when others think about me in such special ways.
I feel truly blessed to have you in my life. I carry
your positive thoughts, love, and support with me
every day. I also want to say thank you to Janis,
Luitgard, and Shelagh for the kind messages you left
in the cards.

I hope you are all doing well and have begun to
enjoy the longer days and the "odd" warm day. It was
so lovely last Sunday; I was able to go for my walk

wearing a t-shirt. I will enjoy my walk later today; however, I think I will need a sweater or jacket.

I miss you all and will look forward to seeing you sometime soon. Again, thank you for touching my heart. I truly do love every one of you!!!

Much love,

Kim

What's Happening in April?

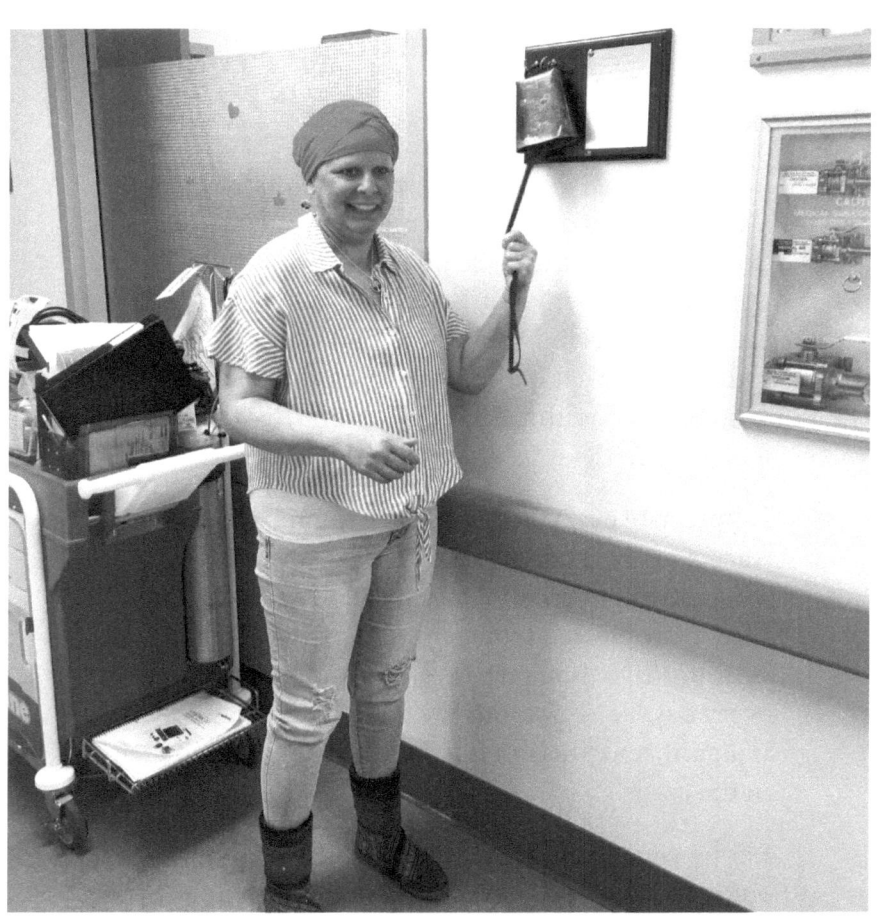

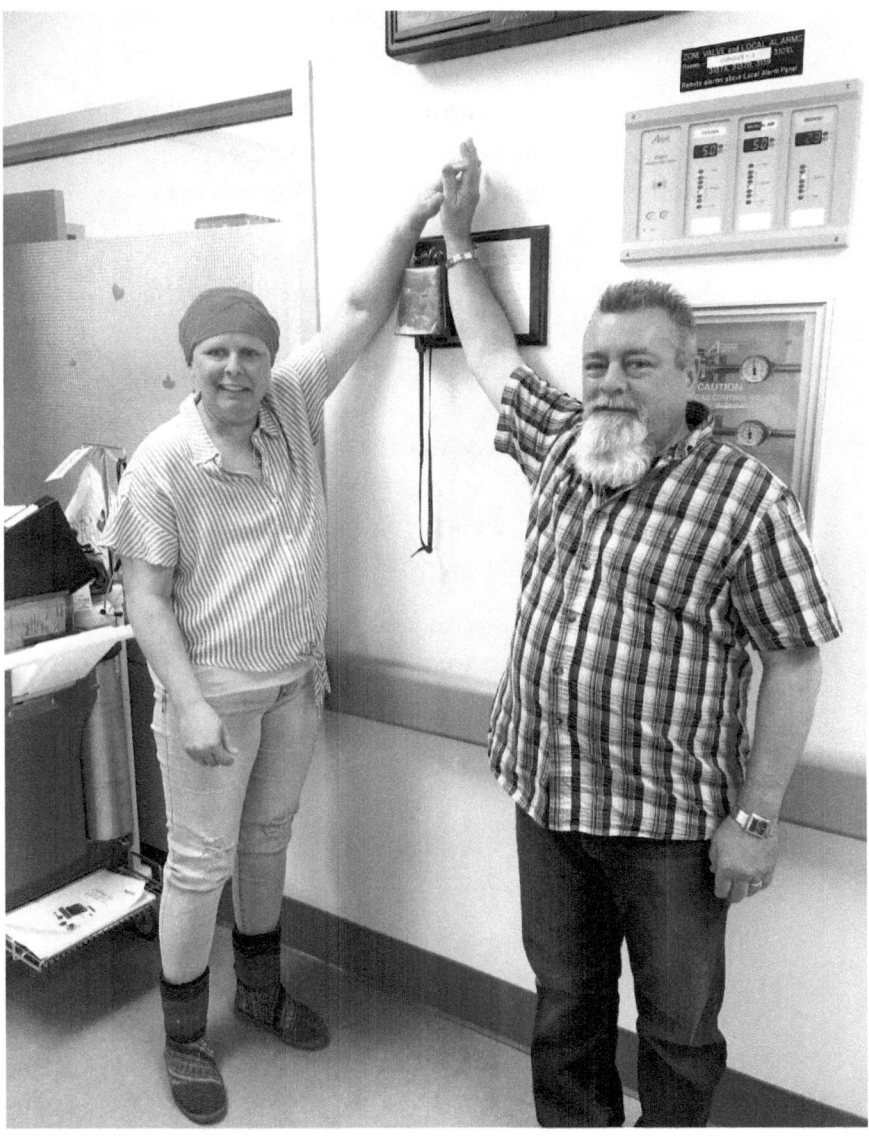

April 8th marked a monumental day in this journey. I completed my last chemo treatment. I cannot express how relieved, elated, and happy I feel. This pic shows my rock, Kevin, and me surrounding the bell. For those who are not familiar with the procedure, when you finish treatments, you ring the bell in celebration.

I will have a few weeks off before radiation begins. I will experience some side effects of this last chemo treatment, but my mantra will be, "This too shall pass, and it will be the last time."

I will look forward to some down time before the radiation begins. I will need twenty-five rounds of radiation, which means I will need to be in Halifax for five weeks. Radiation takes place every day from Monday through Friday. I visited the radiologist department on April 1st to get my tattoos, which are the markings they place to pinpoint where the radiation needs to be targeted.

I have also been fitted with a compression sleeve, which I need to wear on a regular basis during radiation. The sleeve will keep any fluid from building up in my right arm to assist with my lymphedema.

Overall, my spirits are high, and I look forward to the next part of this journey.

This first pic is me ringing the bell. I want you all to know I rang the bell for all of us. I feel surrounded by so much kindness, love, and support from all my family and friends that I felt you with me during this special moment.

I am truly blessed to have wonderful caring people in my life.

Much love

Kim

April 8th

Congrats Kim! This is great to hear! Take care.

Isaac

April 9th

Hey Maria,

Thanks for your cheers yesterday

Kim

May 9, 2019

Dear friends,

I began my radiation treatments on April 29th and will need to have twenty-five in total; sixteen more to go. During the week we live in Halifax at the Lodge That Gives, as I can walk from there to my radiation appointments. Cancer patients stay at the Lodge free of charge and three meals a day are provided. I have experienced some fatigue the past two days; I hit a "wall" yesterday and had to give in and have a nap. Physically I feel so good, so when I feel tired, I cannot figure out why—then my darling husband reminds me I am still going through treatment. Hopefully, I will be finished with these treatments in early June.

So far, my skin is in great shape from the first nine treatments. I am using Lubriderm daily, which need to be applied two to three times per day. The radiation technicians are lovely people. During this journey, I need to state my name and birth date. I hope, when I return to work, I do not introduce myself to someone as "Kim Nelson, February 9th, 1963." I am programmed to state these two facts each time I see someone. Hopefully, I don't say it to a new colleague or parent . . . LOL.

I was excited in April to have my fitting for my prosthetic breast; this was a treasured moment. I have been unable to wear a bra for six months, so this brought some normalcy back into my life. I can not express how sweet Jolene, Family First Medical, was while I was being fitted. It takes special people to do certain jobs and she is well suited for her position. I also will be picking up my swim "boob" tomorrow. Who knew one would need a "regular" and "swim" boob. Sometimes you just gotta chuckle.

I have a few sprigs of hair beginning to emerge. It is unclear now what color is coming in; I keep telling myself it will be blonde, but I think it is looking a little more on the grey tone. Kevin has lovingly coined me his "Chia Pet," which made me crack up. If only I could fertilize my head so that the hair would grow a little more quickly.

If I am able, it is my hope to return to work sometime in June. This, of course, will depend on any side effects I may have from radiation. I am taking this one day at a time and soon it will be over. It is also my hope to share a hallway with you soon!

I hope all is well with all of you. Happy Mother's Day to all the moms—those with human and fur babies.

Much love,

Kim

June 4, 2019, marked the final radiation treatment. My body was fatigued, and my voice had started to fade. Once you are placed on the radiation table, you are required to sit still until the treatment is completed. I had a bit of a cough so I ensured I had a cough drop to suck on with the hopes I would not cough. I made it through number twenty-five and completed my final treatment.

I gave the radiologists a thank-you card for their care and kindness. I was so relieved that the treatment was done. I had a certain area of my skin that burned, and it was painful. I put a saline solution soak on three to four times per day to alleviate the pain.

I was continuing to put forth my positive attitude since my treatments had ceased. I had spoken to a nurse, after one of my radiation treatments, about my concerns moving forward in my life. I had been emoting positivity and could function during my journey, because all I needed to remember was what was happening next. Once treatments were completed, I did not know how to handle the ambiguity of "What is next?" The nurse connected me with four-time cancer survivor, Dr. David McGinley. Dr. McGinley provided candid, sage advice about moving forward. I was grateful for his insights and felt I had some tools to assist me.

This is the letter I crafted for both PRMS and SMES staffs to say thank you:

Dear staff:

Let me begin by saying I acknowledge there are people in the room I have not met and formed a relationship with yet. Please know I include you in my letter because we, at Pine Ridge and St. Mary's are a family. This will be difficult for me to share with you; however, it is important you hear these words from me. I hope I will not cry, but if I do, hang in there because I will get through this on my own.

On September 5th, 2018, I learned I had breast cancer. Maria and Cathy quickly responded by saying, "You take care of you, and we will take care of the school stuff." I cannot express how freeing this statement became as my journey unfolded. The next few months, I was in a whirlwind of appointments, first with the surgeon, then the oncologist, and lastly the radiologist.

During the weeks I came to work, I focused on smiling and tried to fill my day with laughter. I explained to my husband, Kevin, I knew I was stressed; however, the stress was so intense it was both indescribable and immeasurable. As I look back on the first few weeks, I realize I was stumbling about in a shock-filled state only able to regurgitate facts about my diagnosis.

There were days I was crippled with fear when I was driving to work. I would focus on my breathing to help myself calm down before I walked into the building. Once I was in the building, I was embraced by my friends. Thank you for making my days at work, before surgery, as normal as possible before I had to depart. You will never know I much I appreciated your love and support.

After surgery, I felt relief for, to me, the cancer was gone. When we received the pathology news of my treatment plan, we received yet another blow: I would need both chemotherapy and radiation. Since the cancer was also located in my lymph nodes, chemotherapy would be necessary. My state of shock intensified as I consoled my husband who was crying after we received the news. I was so numb during this time; I could not feel my emotions.

Reflecting on the past months since I have been away, I want all of you to know I felt you with me when I was filled with angst, fear, and uncertainty as I meandered through this journey. I was able to endure surgery, chemotherapy, and radiation because I knew I had care, kindness, love, and support from all of you. Each chemotherapy and radiation treatment, I felt your presence lifting my spirits, even on those days I was so scared. I feel I cannot adequately express my gratitude to you for reaching out to me during this time. Every smile, conversation, hug, wink, nod, email, text, food delivery, gift, or visit brought comfort to me in an incredible way. How lucky am I to have received such unconditional love from you, my dear friends.

I have gone into battle with the hope of coming out victorious. I liken myself to a warrior; each warrior comes out of battle with scars both internal and external. Externally, I have evidence of the chemo drug, which leaked out into my arm; a dead vein on my under arm from the wrist to the elbow, bruises from all the blood work the left arm had to endure, a scar where my breast once lived, no eyebrows, eyelashes or hair. I have decided to wear my scars with pride as a sign of a battle well fought. Again, my ability to acknowledge and accept myself is due to the support from you, my army of angels.

This journey also takes you on a path of acknowledging and embracing humility, insecurity, and vulnerability. It was evident as time passed that I needed to let go of any "control" I thought I had during this time. Instead, my focus became a series of following a new schedule: surgery, chemo, blood work, needles, and follow-up appointments.

During my radiation treatment, I was able to meet an incredible man, David, who has battled cancer four times during his life. David is a chaplain and counsels from a religious and personal perspective. David was kind enough to meet with both Kevin and me before my treatment ended. David was blunt with his information to me: I, Kim Nelson, will never be the same person I was before this diagnosis. He told me it will take two years to work through and reinvent myself. I am abundantly aware of the emotional and physical trauma I need to acknowledge so that I can move forward in my life. David told me my journey will be a recreation of Kim 2.0. This experience is life changing. I am different: my views, values, perspectives, and the way I choose to live my life. I have had time to think about what is important and embrace it with the utmost love. May you know and appreciate what you have with the goal of embracing it with your whole heart.

It is my hope you never know this journey, however, if you or someone you love, follows this journey, may they learn what I learned about myself: I am braver than I believed, had faith that I did not know I could fathom, and was stronger than I ever knew was possible.

Going through this journey, I feel an appreciation for everything and everyone in my life. I can liken it to a rebirth; everything feels like I am seeing it for the first time. I am taking everything in, embracing everything and feeling blessed for the experience. I want each of you to know, I shall be forever connected to each of you because of your gracious kindness during one of the most terrifying times in my life. Each of you has helped me more than I can adequately express with words. I am so grateful that our paths have crossed and that your care, kindness, love, and support were given to me unconditionally. I love each of you with all my heart.

SUMMER 2019

My son, James and his wife, Bella, quit their jobs in China to move home to Canada. James was fortunate to get a vacant teaching position at West Kings District High School. James and Bella then bought a car and found a place to live in Berwick. Bella would have to wait to get her working visa, so she worked incredibly hard taking care of their house and baking and cooking excellent meals. I was so thrilled the kids had moved home and that work, home, and vehicle all came together for them.

I visited with family and friends, swam in my pool, hung out in the shade, and felt grateful. Before I knew it, September was around the corner, and I would be going back to work full time.

GETTING BACK TO WORK

I returned to work full time in September and was fortunate to have a counselling intern working alongside me from September to December. Initially I felt elated to be at work—then I had moments of frustration because I could not recall how to use components of the computer program. I did know how to use Tienet and Power School before I left, and my brain froze, and I was stumped on how to use the program. My counselling intern was supportive and kind as I worked through my struggles.

By November, I could feel my emotions becoming dysregulated. I felt angry, bitter, and jealous. I realized I need to reach out for help. Dr. McGinley offered to support me the first year after my treatment. I had amazing, insightful conversations with him on the phone, which helped for a while, then I would begin to experience other difficult emotions, like rage, frustration, and jealousy. I was beginning to get mad that my breast was gone, my arm was hurting, and I did not recognize myself in the mirror. I did connect with Dr. McGinley a few more times, then I decided to figure out how to use the tools he provided to me and move forward.

I had so many thoughts swirling around in my head, so one day I began writing down my journey, which led to this book.

I was battling looking at photos of myself. I knew that girl, yet I did not recognize myself any longer when I looked in a mirror. *Who am I now? How do I move forward?* Months later, I realized I wanted to be the "Kim" before cancer, and I was never going to be that girl again. I slowly began to recognize that I needed to accept I'd had cancer, a scar now marked the right breast area, and I needed to figure out who I was—emotionally, physically, and mentally.

Not only was I struggling with my personal issues, Covid then hit, and we went into lockdown. Being in a helper role, I began to focus on others and what their needs would be during this tumultuous time. It took time before educators would be given directions on how to support our students from home. I was working at a middle school and an elementary school. I was sending fifty or more emails each day to my middle school students and making ten to fifteen phone calls to my younger students. It was tough for me to reach out in this way to our students, but we all managed to get through the best way we could.

I learned in April that my job assignment was changing option one: PRMS-80% and MRHS-20% or SMES-60% and DRES-40%. I had no heads up that any changing was occurring, so I was caught off-guard. During the zoom meeting, I had to ask to leave because I began to cry. I felt frustrated with the option of going to a high school as a 20% position, which would be one day per week. My current position had me 80% at PRMS and 20% and SMES, which is an elementary school. I struggled to meet the needs of the students one day per week at elementary school so I knew how difficult it would be to provide counselling at high school one day per week. I decided to leave a school I loved and had been working at for eighteen years to work at two elementary schools, beginning September 2020. I had had a plan for my retirement; I was going to begin the "retirement purge" from the fall of 2020 through to June of 2023. I had planned to go through my office space and either give resources away, throw them out, or bring them home. This could no longer happen because I now had to go into the school and pack my office and bring everything home.

My note to staff and students to say goodbye:

THE DIFFICULT GOOD-BYE

Dearest PRMS Peeps,

I so appreciated seeing all your faces today. I totally
enjoyed the song; I wish I had recorded it. I had
a good belly laugh and it felt soooo good. I hope
you all have a wonderful, relaxing summer. You all
deserve it! We certainly had some challenging days
the past few months.

I have genuinely enjoyed my time at PRMS, and it is
because of all of you. The atmosphere in the building
has always made me feel safe and secure. You have
all been so supportive over the years when I needed
to get your kiddos. You made coming to work
amazing!!!! I depart with many fond memories,
which I shall hold near and dear to my heart forever.
Your support after my diagnosis was astronomically
phenomenal. I am truly at a loss to find words
to express my gratitude and thanks during that
difficult time.

I had a nice hour-and-a-half-long conversation
with Charm (pronounced Sharm) last week. I feel
at peace because she is going to be a great fit and
asset to the staff and students. We will be talking
again before September to ensure the transition
from one counsellor to another goes smoothly for
our students.

Although I am not sharing physical space with
you, you are now part of my story. A story filled
with great times, friendships, love, laughter, grief,
support, genuine understanding, and compassion.
Departing with these extraordinary memories fills
my heart with joy. The pandemic has proven to me
the importance of staying connected with those we
wish to spend time with and ensuring we make the

time to visit with our friends. I shall sign off with "Be seeing you." Thanks for sharing your smiles with me.

I will miss you.

Dear PRMS students,

This is a difficult letter for me to write to you. I want you to know I am not returning to Pine Ridge Middle School. What I want you to know is how profoundly grateful I am for seeing you, meeting you, and talking with you. I have had many great years working at Pine Ridge Middle School and I shall miss you all dearly.

I will be working at two elementary schools this coming year so I will be helping the Grade 5 students get ready for middle school. Although I will not be in the building everyday, there will be times I will have an opportunity to visit.

It is my intention to be around in the early days once we return to school to make your transition as easy as possible. You will be well cared for with the new counsellor who is coming to support you.

I appreciate you all very much and I will miss you more than I can say. I hope you have a wonderful summer and once we return to school, I will be around to see you in person and ensure you are all taken care of with the new people who will be supporting you.

Much love,

Mrs. Nelson

I continued to provide support to the students I was working with—then reality hit me. I knew I was not going to get the opportunity to say goodbye to students or staff in person due to Covid. The next few months proved to be challenging for me as said goodbye via Zoom to staff and through email to the students. The summer of 2020 was low-key due to restrictions; we could bubble with two people, so Kevin and I bubbled with James and Bella.

WORKING IN SCHOOLS
FROM 2020-2023

The fall of 2020 began with all staff and students wearing masks. Students had to remain in cohorts, which meant all students had to stay together during class, recess, and lunch. Students could not spend time together with or play with other friends who were not in their homeroom. We began social distancing, which meant we needed to stay six feet apart, and students could not share toys or touch anything that belonged to other people. School administrators planned how students would go out for recess and lunch during their free time. At SMES, the property was divided into ten sections and each class was assigned a section and would remain in that area for their free time. The classes would rotate through the ten sections, having a new section each day.

At DRES, three classes went out at a time and were assigned a specific area on the playground they could stay and play in. Each child and staff member needed to ensure they used hand sanitizer when they entered the school building, and hand washing became a regular practice after recess and before lunch to ensure hands were clean. Learning at school certainly became challenging for some of our students, with all the new protocols put in place to ensure our health and safety.

The 2020-2021 school year had learning experiences both in school and at home. We became better equipped to support our students from home although for many families this was challenging. We all managed the best we could to provide fun, educational, well-rounded support, whether it was for academics or for the mental well-being of our students.

Being at two elementary schools, I experienced a huge learning curve. I was petrified when I was around the little ones, primary and Grade 1, for I realized I did not know how to communicate with our little friends. I had an epiphany three months into the school year; I was working with an "adolescent brain," and I needed support. I was used to having conversations with students who were ages 11 – 14 and I realized I was trying to communicate with the elementary students in the same manner and it was not working. I started talking with teachers and listening to how they conversed with their students so I could make changes in how I communicated with the students.

The 2020-2021 school year brought many difficulties, learning opportunities, and the gift of meeting new colleagues and friends.

I began to learn and think differently about supporting students at elementary level. I felt comfort and familiarity with the older students in grades 4 and 5 and realized I needed to change my approach when working with younger students. I began to create resources for hands-on, experiential learning to solidify the counselling work for the children. By June 2021, I began to feel more comfortable and confident supporting our youngest students.

Difficulty arose in May 2021 when my cousin Nancy informed me her cancer had metastasized, and she had tumours on her hip and spine. I was heartbroken and felt like I needed to do something, so I signed up for my first "Run for the Cure" cancer walk, which was to take place in October 2021. I reached out to friends and colleagues and built a team; we would be called Kim's Cancer Crushers. I was recognized for my individual contributions and won first place in the money I raised, and my team won first prize for our collective money raised. Although I know this work did not lessen the pain for my cousin, I wanted the funds raised to go towards metastatic breast cancer research.

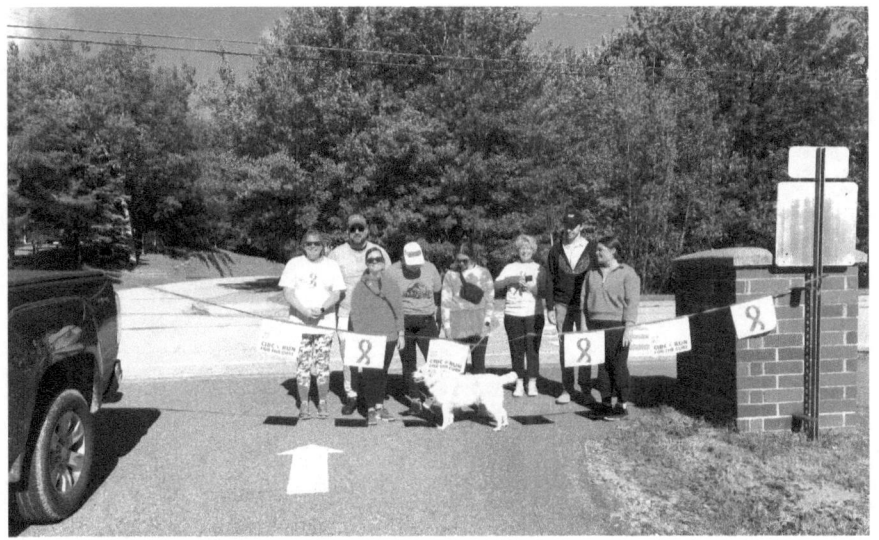

Run for the Cure participants, October 3, 2021. Kim, Isaac, Gillian, Abby, Jen, Cricket, James, Alxys.

We were not able to meet with other teams due to the health protocols put in place during Covid. Our team met in Kingston, and we completed a six-kilometre walk. Before the walk we listened to the song "I Run for Life" by Melissa Etheridge. This song evoked several emotions: gratitude, sadness, fear, and appreciation.

Kim's Cancer Crushers team members and my heroes:

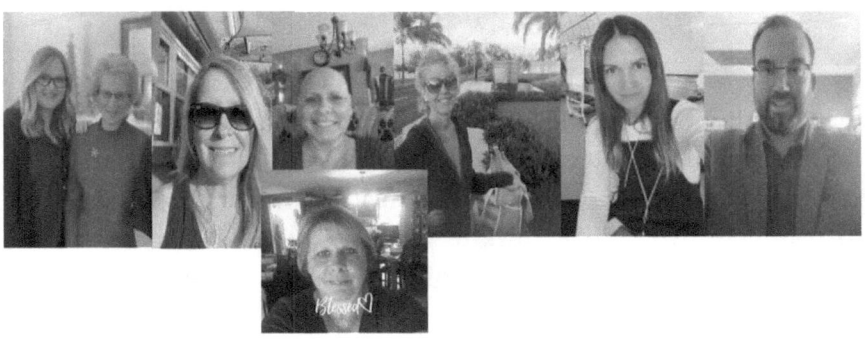

Abby, Lynn, Kim, Cricket, Jenn, Isaac

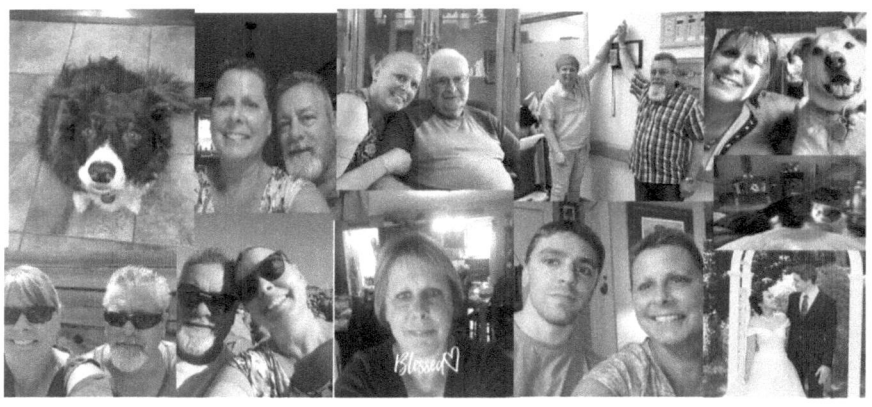

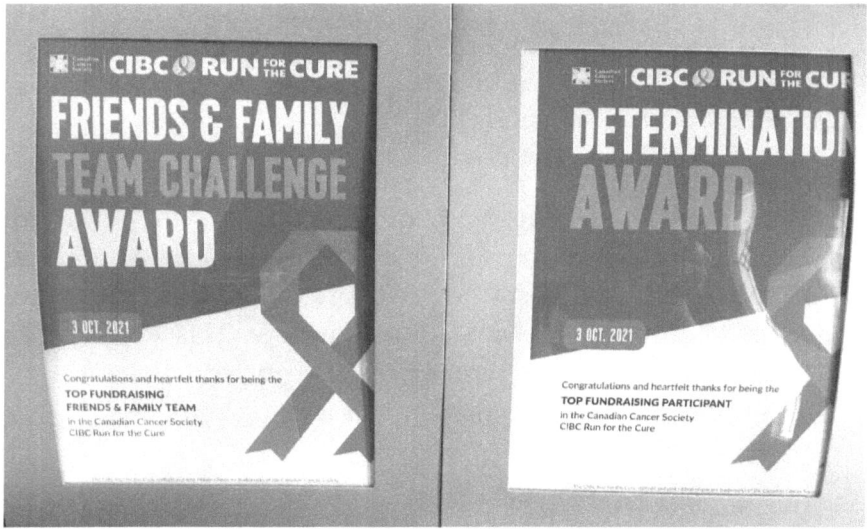

One highlight during the 2020-2021 year was my ability to complete my Master of Education in Inclusive Education. I had had a few setbacks completing this degree. Acadia University allowed me to complete two courses in one year so I could attain my second master's degree. I was so proud of myself for completing work and getting my degree.

Schools during the 2021-2022 school year continued with mask-wearing. Students would eventually have the opportunity to interact with others who were in different classes. Students were again engaged in both in school and at-home learning during this school year. When we returned in January 2022, I presented a Power Point explaining the importance of wearing masks properly. I made the front page of the AVRCE Month Update from a photo taken by our principal, Paula Shehata.

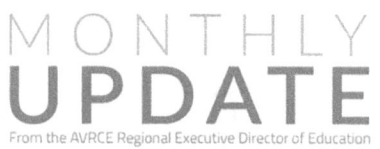
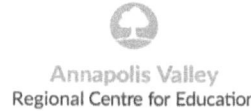
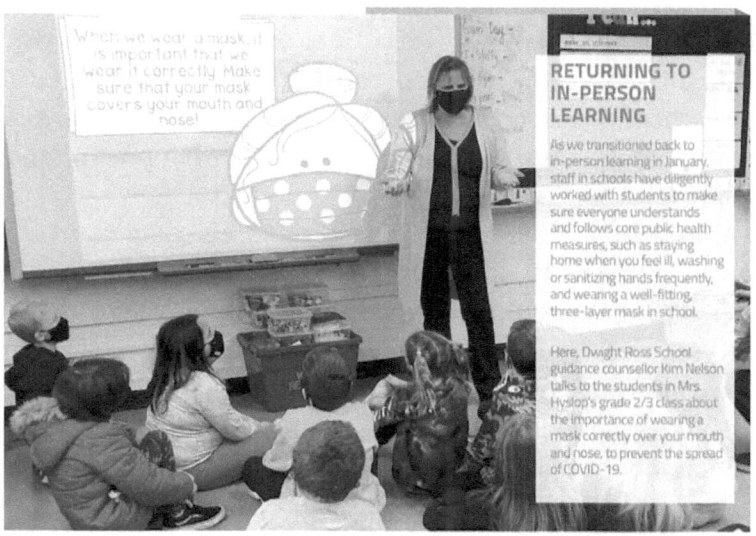

In the fall of 2021, I was fortunate to have an Acadia intern completing her counselling practicum. The intern was a registered yoga teacher, and we discussed the possibility of her offering yoga to our Grade 5 students. She ran two sessions for our students, and I was able to witness their engagement and solace for thirty minutes. Grade 4 students began to ask if they could do yoga too. The intern provided two more thirty-minute sessions for our Grade 4 students. Again, the benefits of this practice became highly evident. I remember thinking I wished I had done the Yoga Tacher Training.

I love it when life presents opportunities and goals can be achieved. All the counsellors in my region had a professional development day, an in-service provided by Blair Abbass and Jenny Kierstead. Blair is a therapist and completed a mindfulness session with us. I was drawn to his voice and the message he was delivering to us. We were focusing on our breathing and embracing calm. Jenny had us participate in a short yoga session demonstrating different poses and asked us to join in if we were able to participate. Since I was in my office, I could complete some of the poses but not all of them. I began to feel connected and drawn to them, as well as a sense of calm during our time together. During the lunch break, I reached out to find out more about the yoga program. I learned I could take the Yoga Teacher Training with a dual certification, which was to begin in March 2022. The dual certification meant I could teach yoga in school but also in private practice. I was sold. I completed the documentation through our professional development fund and was approved.

In March 2022, I began the Yoga Teacher Training course, and I completed it in August of the same year. I am now a Registered Yoga Teacher, RYT. I also took an online course through Yoga Rewind that focused on breast cancer, as well as modification for yoga practice. I worked diligently to acquire my Certified Canadian Counsellor (CCC) credentials with the goal of starting my own practice.

In September of the 2022-2023 school year, I attended wonderful gathering of all school counsellors, along with many others who work within our schools to support the mental well-being of our students. It was heartwarming to be in the presence of others, to embrace and talk in person. I was filled with joy and elation. Through the Yoga Teacher Training, I began setting intentions in the morning. I tried diligently each day to be as present as possible, to ensure I would see and hear things throughout the day that would make me smile or laugh. I also began writing in a gratitude journal. I had written in a journal for a few years, then I stopped. I recalled how much I had enjoyed writing in my journal years ago and thought it was time to add this to my bedtime routine. During the month of February 2023, I wrote the following entry:

1. I am grateful for celebrating my 60th birthday.
2. I am grateful for the beautiful necklace I received from James, Bella and Kevin. The necklace has both the peridot and amethyst birthstones. James and Bella have August birthdays – peridot birthstone and Kevin and I have February birthdays – the amethyst birthstone. I am wearing ALL of us. I absolutely love it.
3. I am grateful for resting last week. I ended up with another cold/flu bug. My body take much longer to heal.
4. I am grateful for the lovely, beautiful conversations Kevin and I have had during the past few weeks. I am so thankful he is in my life.
5. I am grateful for my job. I feel a sense of peace, which in turn is giving me more patience.

On June 8, a retirement banquet was held at Lightfoot in Wolfville. Bella and James accompanied Kevin and me. We had an excellent meal, and I was presented with a gift bag for my service. Our meal was on the ground floor; once we finished our meal, I would walk upstairs to join fellow colleagues who were there to wish me well. I was overwhelmed and overjoyed with all the people who were there to say congratulations. It is difficult to find adequate words to express how happy I felt seeing friends I had not seen in years and catching up with them. I loved the hugs, and my evening was filled with smiles and laughter. I was over-the-moon happy. The first picture shows my DRES family, second picture my PRMS family, and third picture my SMES family.

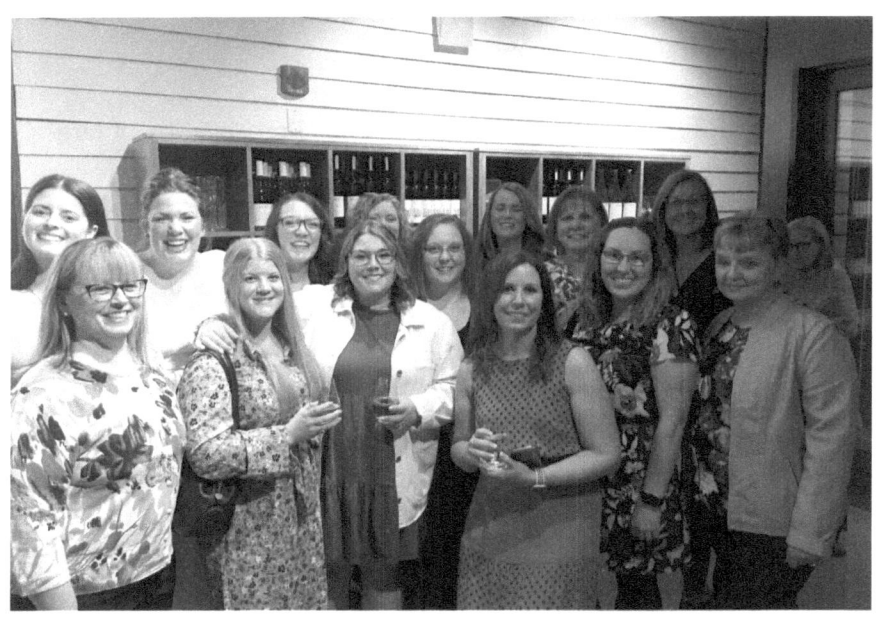

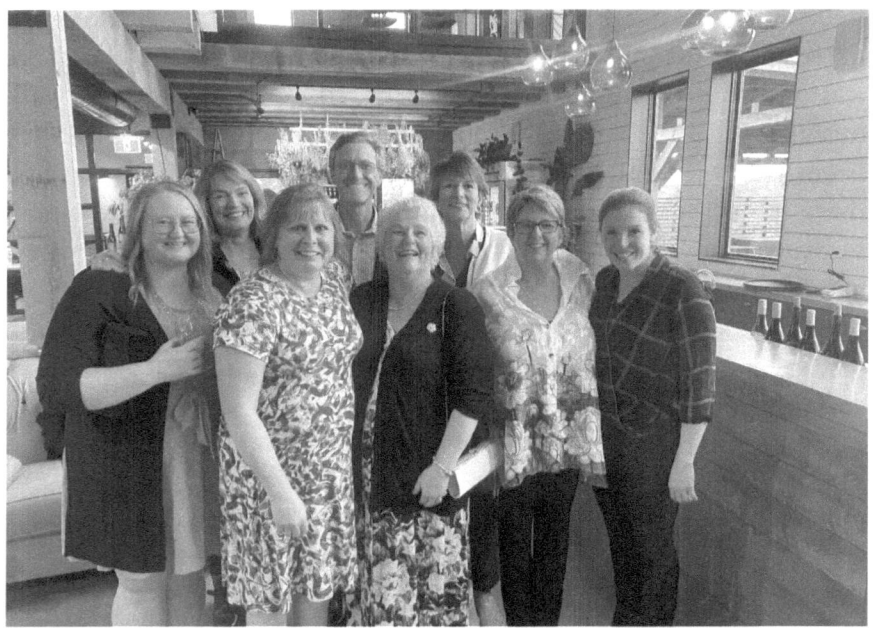

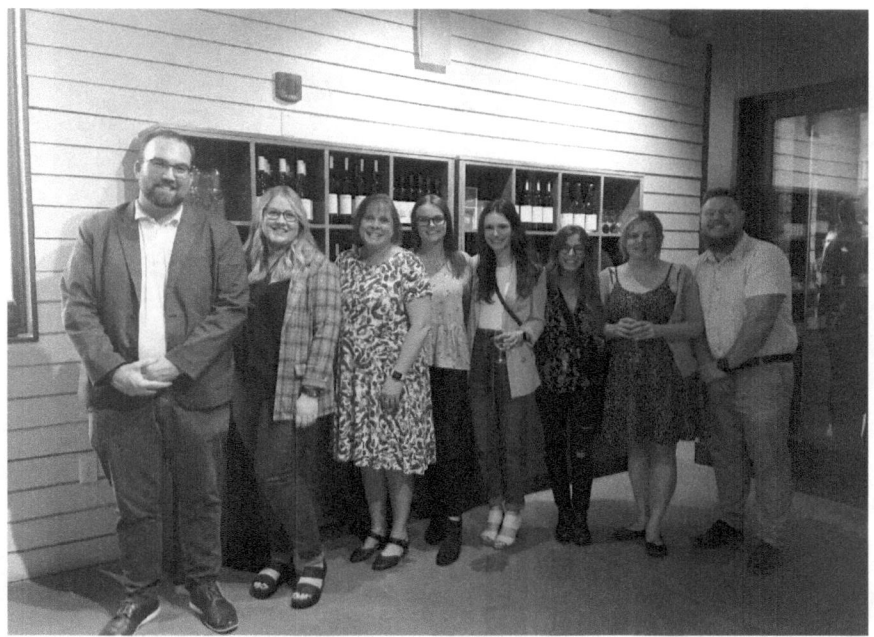

June 30th, 2023 marked twenty-six years working in schools as both a resource teacher and school counsellor. After cancer, it was my expectation that I would work full-time until June 2023. It was important for me to reach this goal. I feel blessed and thankful that I reached this milestone. I had one request as I made my departure. I asked my friends at work for a retirement gift. I asked them to write me a letter or poem about their experience in their teaching career. I wanted to have a keepsake for the days ahead when I will be missing the staff and students. I now have kind messages to help me feel connected to each of them through their words. The two elementary schools I worked at the past three years, 2020 to 2023, gave me a beautiful notebook, scrapbook, and coiled book from Grade 4 students. I was also presented with an award for a "Job Well Done" at our last assembly at SMES. My last day at school, I made my intention to take every moment with appreciation and gratitude. I was able to spend time with some of the students and we shared many laughs and tears. I will cherish the letters and well wishes from staff and students for many years to come.

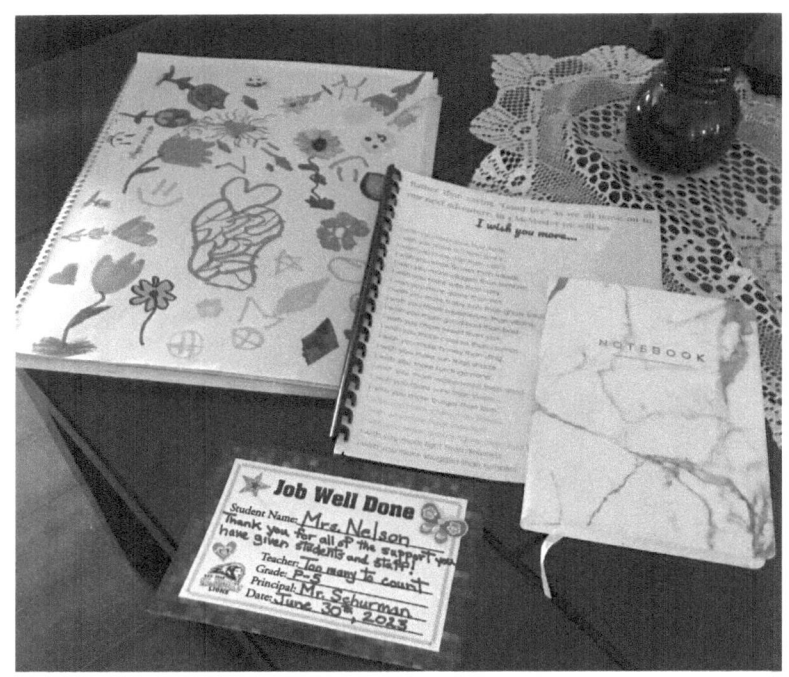

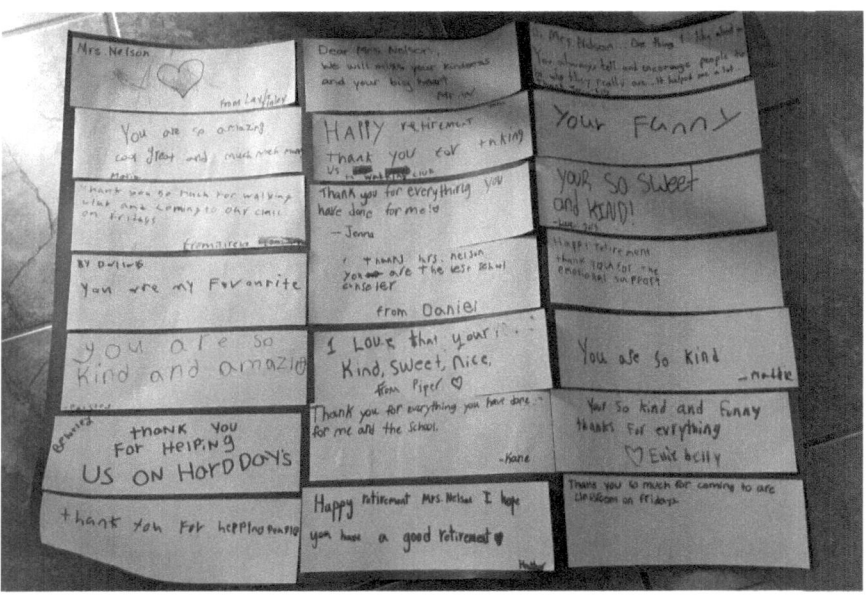

As I reflect on the past five years, I acknowledge how much I struggled. I am abundantly aware of the time, energy, and effort required to do my job
at school. I realized, working full-time since the fall of 2019, I was fatigued and the pain from lymphedema in my right arm had depleted me. I had to come to terms with my new reality, and I continued to work to the best of my ability. I knew when June 2023 arrived, it would be time for me to retire. I left with a happy heart, a feeling of accomplishment, and gratitude for having a career I loved for twenty-six years.

I am excited about the prospects that lie ahead for me. It is my intention to begin my own practice with a specific focus on supporting breast cancer patients and survivors. I am looking forward to what the next chapter brings into my life.

In Loving Memory

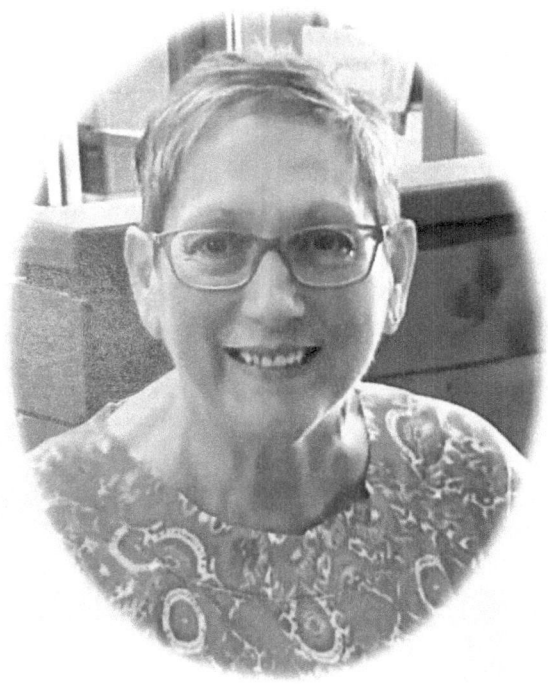

As I was working through the editing process of my book, my dear cousin, Nancy, lost her battle with breast cancer on November 16, 2023. I felt a gut punch and grief unlike anything I have experienced before when losing someone. The reality of this disease hit me hard because my defense mechanisms would not allow me to think that Nancy would die. Nancy and I shared our common journey, and she was "my person" because she utterly understood chemotherapy, radiation, and lymphedema. We jokingly laughed one day and called ourselves, "sleeve sisters."

Nancy's funeral was a beautiful tribute as I listened to stories from her co-workers, her brother, Eric, and the minister. The minister shared with us that Nancy discussed the importance of the following things: when you want to do something, do it, don't wait and take lots of pictures because one day that is all you have left.

Nancy, my dear cousin, I will fondly remember your kindness, compassion, and love. You fought the disease with courage and strength. I will speak of you often and I will look forward to the day when my memories of you make me smile and replace the ache in my heart. I will love, love, love you forever.

Family and friends, your messages to me during my diagnosis helped me dig deep and cope from a place of strength. What I have learned now, your messages brought me comfort when I was grieving Nancy's loss. I appreciate how helpful you have all been to me; your words helped guide me through difficult periods after cancer. I now know the intense power of messages, for you helped me when I needed courage and helped me when I needed comfort.

OUTRAGEOUS LOVE

The messages that follow are from family, colleagues, and friends, which helped me feel connected and hopeful.

September 5

Oh Kim, I am so terribly sad that this is happening to you. I cannot imagine what you and your family must be going through right now. Please know that I am here for you anytime and if there is anything you need from me, please, please just ask me. Promise me you will not worry about anything at school— that's our job. Your job right now is to focus your energies on your health and healing. Sending lots of love.

Xoxo Shelagh Curtis

September 6

Hi Kim.

I was so sorry to hear about your news. Please know that my thoughts and prayers are with you. If there is anything I can do, please let me know.

You are a strong person, but sometimes even the strongest needs a hug and support.

Please know that I'm sending you lots of love
and (((((((((hugs))))))))).

You've got this.

Cynthia Martin

Hi Kim,

I just heard the news. I wanted to let you know I am
thinking of you during this time.

Samantha Harvey

September 7

Kim: I am thinking of you, keeping you in thoughts
and prayers, and I know you've got this. You
are wonderful.

Ashley Rice

Hi Kim, Isaac shared your news with me. Please
know that I will pray for your health and courage in
the days ahead.

Krista Harris

Kim: I am so sorry to hear this news. My wishes and
prayers are with you as you await recommendations
for treatment. May all proceed promptly and offer
you peace of mind.

Love,

Beth Robinson

Kim: I am sorry to hear your health news. I will be thinking of you and sending love and healing to you. Please keep me updated as you progress through this.

My best to you,

Ron Lehr

September 11

Kim: I know that tomorrow is a big day because of your appointment. I'm wrapping you in a big hug and sending lots of love your way.

Shelagh xo

September 12

I cannot imagine what an emotional rollercoaster this must be for you, Kim. I will be ready with an extra-large hug this morning (or anytime for that matter), whenever you're ready!

Xoxo Shelagh Curtis

September 13

Kim: I do not have Lunch Bunch today so if you feel like you'd like a little company or just a quiet place to eat lunch with no one bugging you, come on over!

Shelagh Curtis

September 16

So glad to hear you are taking time for yourself. I will see you tomorrow for sure and you can let me know what you would like to do for Tuesday (re: driving to Wolfville and parking). I was easily able to get into my driveway on Friday by coming up Chestnut and across the first little side street to the right. I had to wait a minute for the steam roller to pass but he let me in. Not sure what tomorrow will bring but I can ask the construction workers at the end of the day when I get home. The side street is always fine for getting in and out—it is just a pain when you actually live on another street and have bags and things to bring in! But even if you came a bit earlier and had to park up there, I could meet you and we could walk in together. Lots of options!

Enjoy the sun!

Shelagh Curtis

September 26

Kim: Thank you so much for the lovely card! That was sweet. Having that chat with you meant a lot to me too. You are such a strong and amazing woman.

I did not get to see you before you left today but I wanted to say good luck at your appointment.

Hailey Milne

September 28

Hi Kim,

I will be thinking of you! Good luck and all the best for what is ahead of you.

Luitgard Budd

September 30

Hi Kim,

I am waking up to your letter and am filled with so many different emotions. I can only imagine that this must have been incredibly difficult to put down on paper. I have said this before but I'm here for you in any way that you need.

You are such a support to all of us at school and we're so grateful to have you in our lives. Thank you for putting your faith in us and sharing this update with us. Know that you are surrounded by *outrageous love* and positive energy every day.

Shelagh Curtis xoxoxo

Hi Kim,

Just wanted to let you know that you are in my thoughts and prayers.

Love,

Beth Robinson

October 1

Hi Kim, I feel truly privileged that you are sharing this. I am not particularly good at words of support and encouragement, but I wish you the best in your recovery, my and my family's thoughts will be with you. I know we do not know each other well, but I do live in Berwick, and if there is anything you need or that I could help you or your family out with please let me know.

Take care, Shane MacDow

Kim: I am so sorry to hear that news. I believe that if attitude has as much to do with successful outcomes as the professionals say, then you have that part down. Use your personality and obvious love for your family to aid in your road to success. I wish you the best of luck and will keep you in my thoughts.

- Emily Wheeler

Kim: I am sending positive energy your way! So sorry that you received this news, but glad that the doctors are acting fast. I wish you well on your surgery and your recovery. You are a strong person!

Keep in touch!

Erin Langille

Hi Kim, I have been thinking about you. I am so sorry to hear these results.

You are strong, kind, and determined—you will get through this. I am sending you the biggest hug ever and positive thoughts for a successful recovery.

D. Fitzgerald

Oh Kim, I am so sorry to hear about this diagnosis. I will be thinking of you through this challenging

time. Sending healing, calming energy and support
from afar.

Laura

Thank you for updating us. My thoughts are with
you, and I am sending healing and positive vibes
your way. Take care. Xo

Andrea Baker

Hi Kim—I am sad to hear about your diagnosis.
It does sound like you are well cared for. I had a
wonderful time hanging out with you as well—you
are very inspirational professionally and personally.
Please stay connected and let me know how
everything is.

Take care,

Nicoline Hussey

Kim: I am so sorry you are going through this. But
you are a strong, resilient woman, and you have this!
I am sending you lots of love and healing vibes right
now, but especially on October 18. I know you have
a strong support system, and they will help you get
through this.

I wanted to pass on a contact for my naturopath
in case you are interested. Perhaps you know her
as she's located in the valley . . . it's Dr. Lois Hare.
She is PHENOMENAL and has helped various
family members through many medical conditions,
including breast cancer. The medical system will

take good care of you I am sure, but Lois will help you do extra things to make your body as healthy as it possibly can be while you fight this. Worth looking into—so I will paste her contact info below.

Take care,

Beth Noel

Hi Kim,

I am deeply sorry to hear about the results. Here is a shocking but positive thought for you . . . my mom and four of her sisters have all been diagnosed with breast cancer in the past and they are all alive and healthy today :). Best wishes for you and a speedy recovery.

Tracy Beaton

October 17

Hi Kim.

I just wanted to let you know that I have been and will continue to say an extra prayer for you and the surgeons tomorrow. May God be with you and guide the surgeons' hands. It is no fun having surgery, and I cannot even imagine how you must be feeling.

If there is anything I can do, please do not hesitate to ask. Hang in there. Sending lots of love and positive vibes your way.

Cynthia Martin

October 19

Hi Kimmy Gibbler,

Jack and I are thinking about you and if there is anything we can do at any time do not hesitate.

Kelly Saunders

October 23

Kim: I am not sure if you will be checking this email. I hope that you are not because I don't want you to be doing any work. I just wanted to say that I admire you for healing through this unbelievably challenging time by writing a note to the staff. You are an incredibly brave and generous person to give your precious and positive energy to us when you need it so much for yourself.

I know we are all thinking of you, and I hope you feel that, especially on the hard days.

Stay in touch and wrap yourself in all the love that I know is coming to you.

Rest, and do not worry about anything here. It will all be here when you are ready for it.

Jill Gidney

Xo

October 24

Hey Kim!

Thinking of you! I know you are probably very sore, but I am sending you a virtual hug . . . that way it can be as hard or soft as needed! Feel free to use this

hug any time! I love the note you sent to the staff . . .
it will be nice (believe it or not) to have these details
in time to come to look back on.

Have a wonderful sunny day!

Sue Kennie

October 25

Hi Kim,

Thinking of you. . .. wishing you all the best for
a speedy recovery! Please let me know if you
need anything.

Love,

Cathy Matheson

October 26

Kim: I just wanted to let you know that I think of
you often. I hope you are taking care of yourself and
getting well. And that Kevin and the puppies are
doing well too. Sending you positive vibes!

Love Hailey

November 8

Hello Kim,

I read your update letter and just wanted to let you
know that my family and I have you in our thoughts
and prayers. The positivity and strength you have
displayed throughout this time have been admirable

and a reflection of your amazing character. I truly hope that if presented with an obstacle like the one before you now, I possess a fraction of the bravery and gumption you have displayed.

I have been here now at PRMS for ten years and not having you present in the school is something I have yet to get comfortable with. As my levels of comfort are of paramount concern here on the second floor, I highly recommend you get well and get your ass back at Pine Ridge.

All the best and take care. Thoughts with you and yours,

Clint Bungay

November 9

Cathy said you're coming in for lunch!!! Soooooo happy!!! Get ready for a deluge of hugs from everyone!

Shelagh C

November 12

Thanks, Kim.

Good to get your news which sounds incredibly positive. Best of luck with the continuing treatment. Thanks for keeping us in the loop. We are rooting for you.

Warm regards,

Mike Corbett

Kim: It is wonderful to hear from you! Thanks so much for the update. It is good to know that surgery went well and that you have a plan in place for the next steps. This is not a club that anyone wants to join, but I am glad to know that you have got the "initiation" out of the way. It is hard to believe that you are already four weeks post surgery.

Take good care of you. Hugs to you and Kevin.

Love, Beth Robinson

Yay . . . so happy to hear you are healing well and beating all your "benchmarks."

I still hope to get down to visit before the real holidays set in. I am sending lots of warm hugs your way and tremendous positive energy. Take good care of yourself.

Lynn Aylward

November 20

Hi Kim,

I had no idea about your health challenges. Sending you lots of love, hugs and prayers. Please let me know if you need anything at all. May all the love and compassion you give to others be radiated back to you. I'm here if you need anything.

Take care,

Bernice MacNeil

November 28

Kim: Just thinking about you this morning! I wanted to tell you what a wonderful surprise it was to see you at school yesterday. Seeing you always puts a spring in my step!

I am not sure what your schedule is like over the next week, but I was wondering if you might be up for another short visit if I popped by after school? I am sure you have a ton of visitors, and I don't want to interfere with that. No pressure and you do not need to let me know right away.

Missing you heaps. Big, big hugs,

Shelagh xoxo

December 11

Hey Girl,

Just dropping you a line to let you know that Jack and I are thinking of you and to send you a few Christmas jokes.

Kelly Clause

December 15

Hi Kim,

I believe my advent gift for you was today. I have it already fresh tonight and would love to drop it off to you tomorrow if there is a time you will be home. If you opened it, you know what I am talking about. Hehehe. Let me know what works.

Candice

December 18

Dear Kim,

I thought a lot about you last week. And sent positive thoughts your way. I am sure you are glad your first treatment is over so that you know what to expect. How did Kevin do?

I am on forced rest as I fell down the bottom stair and broke my foot yesterday. I am really annoyed because the house was not quite finished being decorated and have not baked a thing. Oh well, soon the family will be here, and baking can be part of what we do together. As I always say, bake early; bake often. It gets eaten about as soon as it comes out of the oven anyway.

I hope the treatment went well and the aftereffects are manageable.

Thinking of you,

Sheri

December 21

Good morning, Kim:

I really appreciate your enthusiasm, especially in tough times. You are such an encouragement! I just to let you know that I have been praying for you and Kevin, especially as your treatments were approaching and last Thursday especially.

Have a wonderful Christmas!

Stacy

December 24

Hi Kim,

I have been thinking about you everyday and wondering how you have been feeling. Your cousin's passing would have been so difficult to cope with at any time, but with Christmas so close, and at a time when you are trying to focus on staying calm and strong because of your own health challenges, this must be incredibly difficult for you. I am sorry that you are having to go through all of this. I suspect that you will find a bit of quiet time to celebrate her life and the person she was, in your own way, and in your own time.

Other stuff:

Last day of school went pretty well. Not too many meltdowns overall—the kids were just really excited, as were the teachers. I did not end up going to Maria's house because our boys (and one girlfriend) were coming up, and we also had to go out to another even—my husband's cooking group was throwing a get-together over at the Malt House in Grand Pre. It was a really fun evening with fantastic food, but I had other events the previous two nights (too much for a school week!!!) and I was super exhausted the next day. But then . . . we geared up again the next day to celebrate Liam's twenty-seventh birthday bash here on Saturday! We prepared for all day and again, it was loads of fun, but I ended up going to bed early and let the young people carry on! Yesterday was a much more restful day: we ate leftovers, went for walks, I did some knitting, and we talked. Our youngest son, Noah, went to the airport last night to pick up his girlfriend, but they were not back until very late, so I'll see her today when she wakes up.

Today: we will have another quiet day of walking, hanging out together, playing music and singing. It is lovely to have cooler weather even though there's no snow. Those warm, rainy days felt weird. As for dinner tonight, I think we all voted on homemade pizzas and salads, so I'll get the dough ready this morning and we'll all help to make them later on. Liam's girlfriend will head back to her family this afternoon (Dartmouth) and Noah's girlfriend, Hope, will stay with us. She is from Vermont, but she just met up with her mom, brother and stepdad this past week in Montreal for Christmas.

I am not sure how tired you've been feeling, but hopefully you have enough energy to doing your regular walks—good for the body, good for the mind. I want to wish you the loveliest of holidays with Kevin, family and friends this week. Soak up all those beautiful lights and music and know that I'm thinking of you every day.

Sending you love and big, big hugs,

Shelagh xoxo

December 29

Kim,

Wishing you, Kevin, and James and his partner all the best in 2019. May health and happiness be the backdrop to all of the events in your lives in the year ahead.

Love,

Beth

January 12

Hello my dear,

I have been thinking about you every day and just wanted to say hi. I am hoping that your energy level has returned to a good level since your last chemo treatment—I keep a picture in my mind of you walking down to the convenience store and back most days. Last time you wrote, you talked about the next hurdle of hair loss, and I have been wondering how you're coping with that. I remember you talking about how you might look without your hair and so you tied it all back one day just to see. I suspect that when it happens it's very different from what you'd imagined—others can't possibly know how it feels unless it happens to them. I understand that this is all part of your "journey", but I desperately wish I could do something for you to make all this crap go away. Because I am unable to do that, I am sending you a massive, virtual bear hug. Hope you can feel it.

I do not have any interesting news to share with you, so I'll just let you know what I'm up to. Right now, I can hear the wind outside and I know the temperature is a bit scary . . . I may *not* do a walk today! Jeff and I are trying to walk most days and we are also back on our Paleo diet, which kind of took a backseat with my mom and dad's difficulties. I already feel more energetic and calmer in my mind.

That is partly due to me "drawing a few more lines in the sand" and working hard to carve out more time to do the things I love to do. I am reading and knitting more, I started a rug hooking project (I'm using some of my mom's rug hooking wool that I brought back with me, which she would have loved), and Jeff and I signed up for another yin yoga class. I think you would really love this type of yoga, Kim. It is a gentle, restorative, AND also uplifting practice. My yoga instructor has given me a few names of reputable instructors down your way, if you're ever interested.

Over the Christmas holiday, I came to a few conclusions; one of them is that with the never-ending demands of the teaching profession, I can realistically only handle another few years of this constant energy drain. There is no longer any "off button" and I (like many other teachers) have a hard time saying *no*. So, I will start to look into the whole retirement things and think about what else I'd like to do. I am not ready to stop working, but I know that I need to think about a change. I have not told anyone at work. The decision is both freeing and a bit scary—but when I think about all the big things Jeff and I have done, those have ended up being the most rewarding experiences in the end. I think that when you take any leap of faith you cannot help but grow and learn a lot about yourself and what you're capable of. I'll keep you posted.

I may drive into Halifax tomorrow to buy a few pairs of footwear on sale. My foot problem is ongoing and with the exception of my new running shoes (post orthotics), and my old Keen boots and Keen shoes, I packed up my other shoes/boots last week and gave them all away. I kept hoping I would be able to wear them again but having them staring back at me in my closet was just making me feel "stuck" and frustrated—it actually feels better to have accepted the situation and to move forward. Now if only good quality shoes weren't so expensive!!! Yeesh!

Nothing much else going on. I will write again very soon, but please take good care in the meantime.

Sending loads of love,

Shelagh xoxo

January 15

Hi Kim,

I am glad to hear that you are tolerating your chemo treatments well and that you are doing little things around the house!

You are not missing much in this cold snap outside—I went for a walk last night and have a lovely red wind-burnt hue to my face today!! I will be twenty weeks this Thursday, and I go for my ultrasound on Friday to make sure everything is going according to plan in there! We are not planning on finding out the sex, though—that will be a surprise at the end of the road.

I hope things continue to move along fairly smoothly, and that your energy will start to come back soon after these treatments are done!!

Ashley Rice

January 16

Kim: You sound in good spirits in spite of this recent round of chemo and the hair loss. I have been thinking a lot about learning to be comfortable with who you are and what you look like at any given time (make-up or no make-up). We should all be trying to take a page out of your play book and learn to live more deeply and honestly. It is interesting how much power we allow society to have over us, to dictate how we should dress, how we should look, etc. Your experience has been a humbling one for me, and I am working to make some changes in my own life as a result.

As for crocheting, I have not done it since I was ten years old! But if you ever feel like hanging out to crochet for a while and want some company, I could bring my knitting! Just let me know!

Today is a half-day. Normally, I have so much paperwork to get through that I cannot get excited about sitting through an unhelpful/useless P.D. session. But today, the teachers are meeting in their groups to work on goals (I think?) and CORE will meet briefly for a half hour, then I am able to get started on my West Kings transition notes. So excited to have some time to get a start on them!

I can imagine you all curled up with your puppies keeping you warm during this cold snap! The temperatures sure make it harder to get out walking—I have only walked a few times in the past week. I know I need to make more of an effort, but I don't have proper (warm) footwear because of my foot issue. I went to look for boots last weekend in

Halifax but none of the boots felt comfortable on that foot . . . sooooooo frustrating. I'm also not a fan of shopping malls so the whole trip felt like a waste of time, gas, energy, etc. I'll have to do some more online investigation, I think.

Alright, I need to get moving and pack up my lunch, get organized (ie. find my car keys—drives Jeff crazy!). Stay warm today and do some lovely things for yourself: hug your dogs, listen to some beautiful music or an uplifting podcast, eat nourishing food, and think about all the love people are sending your way!

Talk with you soon,

Shelagh xoxo

January 24

Hi Kim,

Here is a video that will brighten your day; we are always thinking of you.

Miss You

Love Mark, Kim & Jen

xo

January 26

Hi Kim,

Hoping you are enjoying this beautiful sunshine today; it is nice to look at even in the house. :) Koda, my dog, has been loving the sun today as she has twice been out to play frisbee. She has yet to realize that we do not enjoy playing frisbee when it's minus 20 outside. If we only shared her passion for sport in freezing temps.

All is well at school—at least for our 8s. I told them after being in the office one day that I was so happy to be back with them as they were so normal compared to the other grades lol. I am lucky to have such a kind group.

I am so excited to see the longer daylight hours. It will be March before we know it and we will be looking forward to seeing flowers. I cannot wait! Janice Ring mentioned on FB that she was raking her lawn, and I must say I was a tad bit envious.

Just wanted to check in to say hi and that you are never far from mind. Take care of yourself and I hope to see you soon!

Take care,

Cindy

February 2

Hi Kim,

We are glad your treatment went well. The mitts and hat look so nice on you. You look great! I found another video to give you a good laugh.

Always thinking of you.

Love Mark, Kim & Jen

Xoxo

February 3

So glad you are feeling positive. I cannot believe I missed seeing you again. Glad we got to chat the other day. Take care!!

M

Hi Kim,

I just read your update. It is nice to hear from you and I am sending lots of thoughts and prayers and hoping for only the best for you and your family.

Please know that you are often mentioned at the school and people are asking questions around your recovery and the students are wondering about how you were doing as well.

All the best, Isaac

February 5

Hi Kim,

Glad to read that most everything has been positive to date! You are a true fighter.

I am always thinking of you and always sending hugs and best wishes your way!

Take care and hang in there!

Ann Marie C

February 11

Hi Kim,

Thank you so much for forwarding the updates and keeping me in the loop. It was lovely to see you–your resilience is inspiring.

I am at your wonderful school today to offer extra support. Your presence on Thursday brought such comfort to the staff...what an amazing gesture. I am so glad we had a chat and chance to catch up.

Take good care and know that I am thinking of you.

—

Paula Guy, CCC

February 24

Hi Kim,

Mark had a cold this week, he will call you tomorrow. Glad to hear you got the card, thank you for sending the picture, so good to see you.

We are happy you are feeling good. We think about you every day.

Mark, Kim & Jen

February 24

Sorry to hear your chemo was delayed until tomorrow because of a low white count. As frustrating as this must be, your decision to change how you view the hiccups and hurdles that come your way will definitely help make those disappointments a little more bearable. Hang in there. Is this your fourth chemo treatment? I have no idea if time feels like it's going quickly for you or not these days, but I'm hoping you have enough projects (and sufficient energy to work on them) to help occupy your mind in between treatments.

I attended a knitting workshop on Saturday with my friend from NB. It was lovely to see her, and we both learned a lot. I kept thinking the whole time about the "Brain Gym" exercises I do with my morning Resource students—I was trying to learn how to do stranded knitting with yarn in both hands! Talk about a steep learning curve! It felt like learning how to write with my left hand! It is going to take some time to get the hang of it, but it's a much fast way to do stranded knitting than what I was doing before. Patience and practice! The practice I can do . . . not sure if you know this, but patience is not my strong suit! I have attached a picture below of the mitten I started.

Jeff and I are continuing to sort and purge whenever we have an hour here and there. We are doing really well, and it sure feels good—I'm both embarrassed and thrilled to admit that I finally sorted through our last New Zealand Vanlines moving box!!! We moved here in 2007 but started our first move overseas to Australia in 2000 . . . I have just never really had time to stop and catch my breath long enough to catch up with our lives and new jobs. Some very exciting years, but way too many new jobs in the past nineteen years. I would not recommend it.

I talked with my dad today and he sounded really good—no short-term memory, as usual, but cheerful, he knew who I was, and he asked about Jeff and our boys. I miss him. I am hoping to get back in April for a couple of days to help out a little bit with some of his appointments before I see him again in the summer.

Just looking at the weather forecast—sounds like a carbon copy of the past few storms! Crazy! I am so glad that Kevin is able to drive you to your appointments when the roads aren't great. We have had some sloppy driving at times, but we've been fortunate in that they've given us storm days. I have lost track of how many (too many) but it's out of my control.

Phys Ed assessment tomorrow and Tuesday (weather permitting) for one of our gr. 8 students, and we also have our West Kings transition meeting as well as all of our gr. 5 transition meetings with the feeder schools this week. Busy week!

That is about it for now. Take good care until my next email.

Love and hugs,

Shelagh xoxo

February 28

Hi,

So sorry to hear about Bear, we know the loss is terrible. Will be talking with you soon. Miss and think of you everyday.

Will call you on Sunday, the squares look yummy!

Love

Mark

March 4

Dear Kim,

I had a dream about you the other night and when I awoke, I realized that my brain was reminding me that I had not been in touch for a while.

I hope that all is going well for you and that your energy is increasing as we move into the longer days of approaching spring.

Say hi to Kevin and take good care!

Love,

Beth

March 5

Oh Kim, I am so very sorry to hear your news about Bear—my heart is aching for you, Kevin and James. Jeff and I are "dog people" too and know only too well the loss of a beloved pet. I imagine that losing Bear at such a challenging time in your own lives must be that much more heartbreaking. I have no doubt that Bear gave you as much love as he received from you, and in the end, I'm not sure any of us can hope for more than this from life. Please know that I'm wrapping you and Kevin in a big hug and sending peaceful thoughts your way.

As sometimes happens in life, as one door appears to close, another opens: the news of James and

Bella's move must feel like a birth, and I am thrilled that you're getting this news now! You are such a close family and I suspect that James has really been missing you both. Get excited for June!!! Cannot wait to hear all the news—where will they live, jobs, etc . . .

As for your next big step, radiation, I had no idea that you would require so many treatments, but I am relieved to hear that you have a lovely place to stay in Halifax. I am hoping we can see each other briefly before you start that treatment, but I understand if you have to be careful about being around others in case, we compromise your immune system. Let me know if you think a visit might be a possibility.

No news from my end other than drowning in IPP and resource reports—counting the minutes until they are finished. Such an enormous "time and energy sucker" and I am having a hard time justifying the countless hours/weeks that go into them. Many of my parents struggle to read them and many of them cannot be bothered. Argh!!!!

Okay, enough of that! I will write again very soon and will be thinking of you in the meantime.

Sending lots of love. Take good care.

Shelagh xoxo

March 6

Hi Kim!

Happy soon-to-be Spring! Think how we were discussing March as being way off in the future a few months ago and now here we are! I am so happy you have just a couple of chemo appointments left. What you described sounds so unpleasant; I wish I could make it better for you. I am hopeful that the sun will shine, and you will feel its warmth and know that all this will end, and we will soon be able to enjoy Pepsi by the pool. I promise I will not be complaining at all this summer of the heat . . . I will happily sweat out 30-degree weather and be glad I do not need a sweater.

It was lovely to hear from you. I hope you will feel up to a visit soon. Take care of yourself as you are a very special Panther! :)

Cindy

March 7

Hi Kim,

Thank you for your letter. It is great keeping us in the loop as we think of you often. I wanted to pass along my condolences for the loss of Bear. It is never easy, even when we know they have lived a full, long life. Thoughts are with you.

Hugs,

Candice

March 8

Hi Kim,

I have to say, it was tough reading your update . . . I just feel so sad for you . . . cannot imagine the tough days and the frustration.

Then, to lose Bear . . . but it sounds like he was given so much love right to the end—you could not have given him a better life!

I am hoping that once we can get rid of this winter weather and we have longer days with more sun, that this will help give you a lift and make the days seems a bit better.

Take care, stay strong, and I hope every day you feel better.

Ann Marie C

June 14

Thanks so much for the updates! You are one beautiful, resilient, courageous woman and I feel so fortunate to know you:)

Let us plan to meet up at the end of August when it will be fresher for you to start the school year. I am not far so we can always meet again, if necessary, in September.

Take good care!

Paula Guy

It is my hope you never know this journey. If you are diagnosed with breast cancer, may you experience the comfort, compassion, and outrageous love that I received during my most difficult life challenge. May you also learn about your courage and strength from within.

I am here for you. If you need a friend who has been on the journey, please feel free to send me a message via email: nelson536987@gmail.com or reach out through my private counselling practice: Hope and Strength from Within Counselling Services. I am located on Psychology Today; here is my link: https://www.psychologytoday.com/ca/therapists/hope-and-strength-from-within-counselling-services-aylesford-ns/1168461

Here are cherished pictures I took over the journey. I am at peace with my past, have accepted the changes that occurred during my cancer journey, and enthusiastically embrace the future with an open heart.

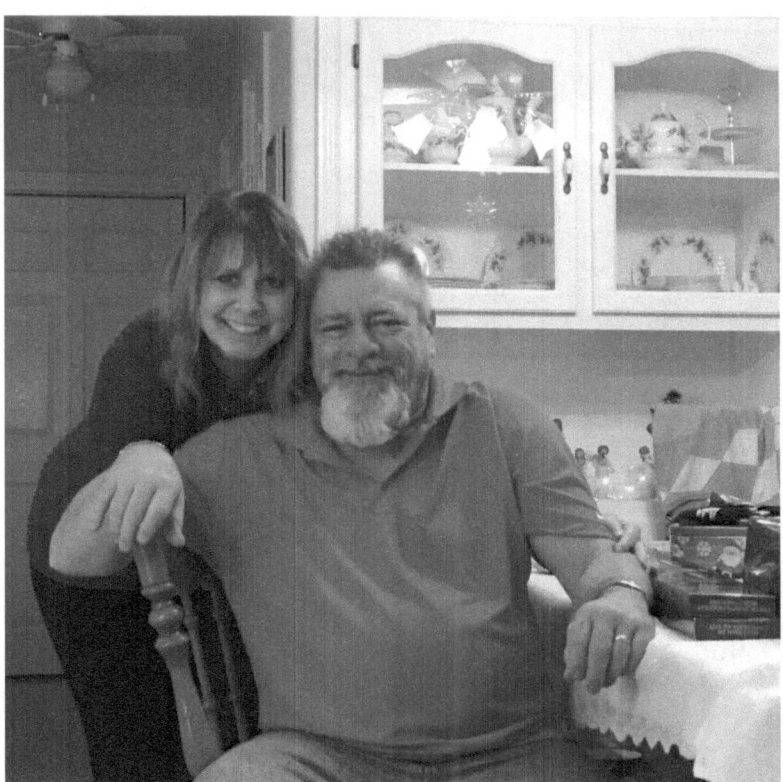

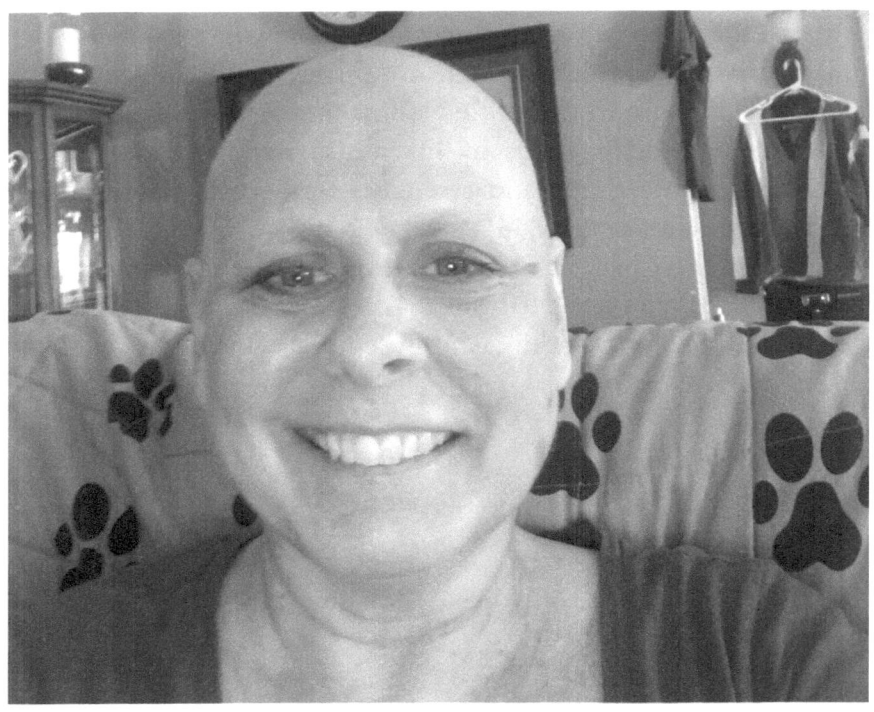

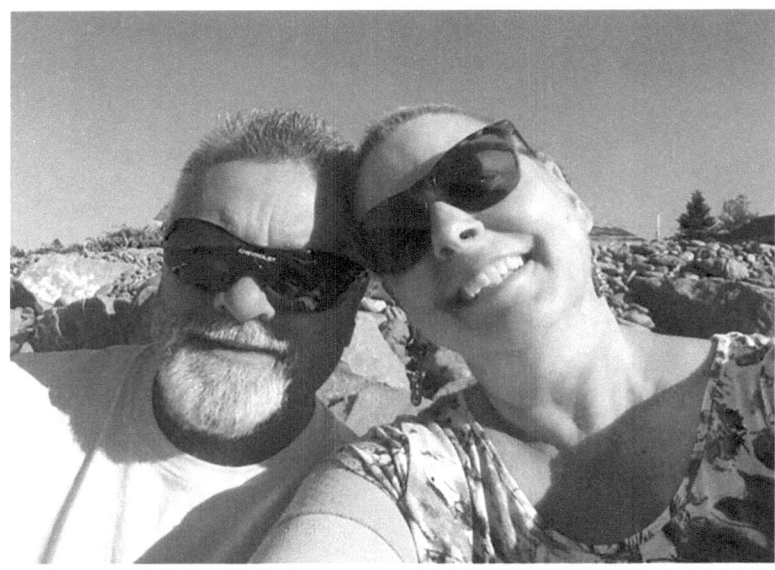

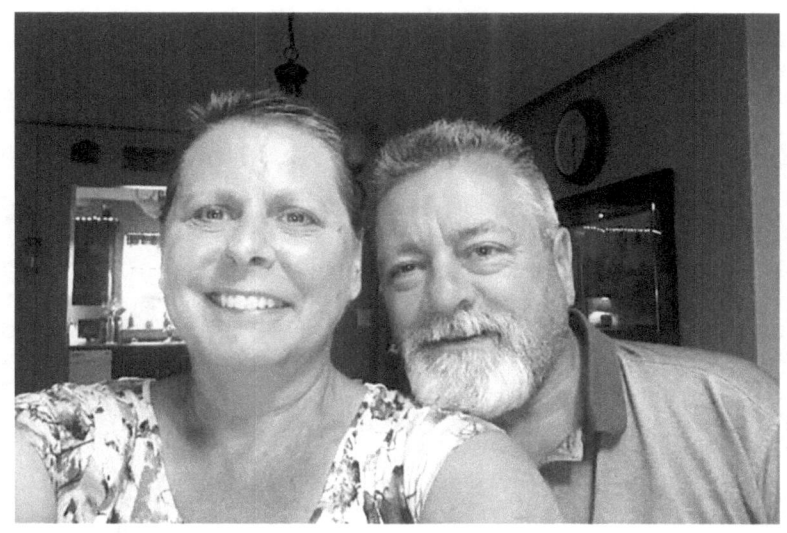

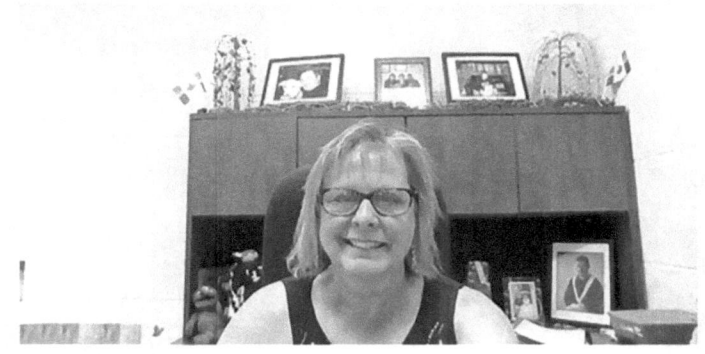

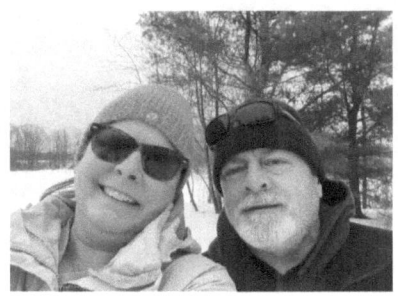

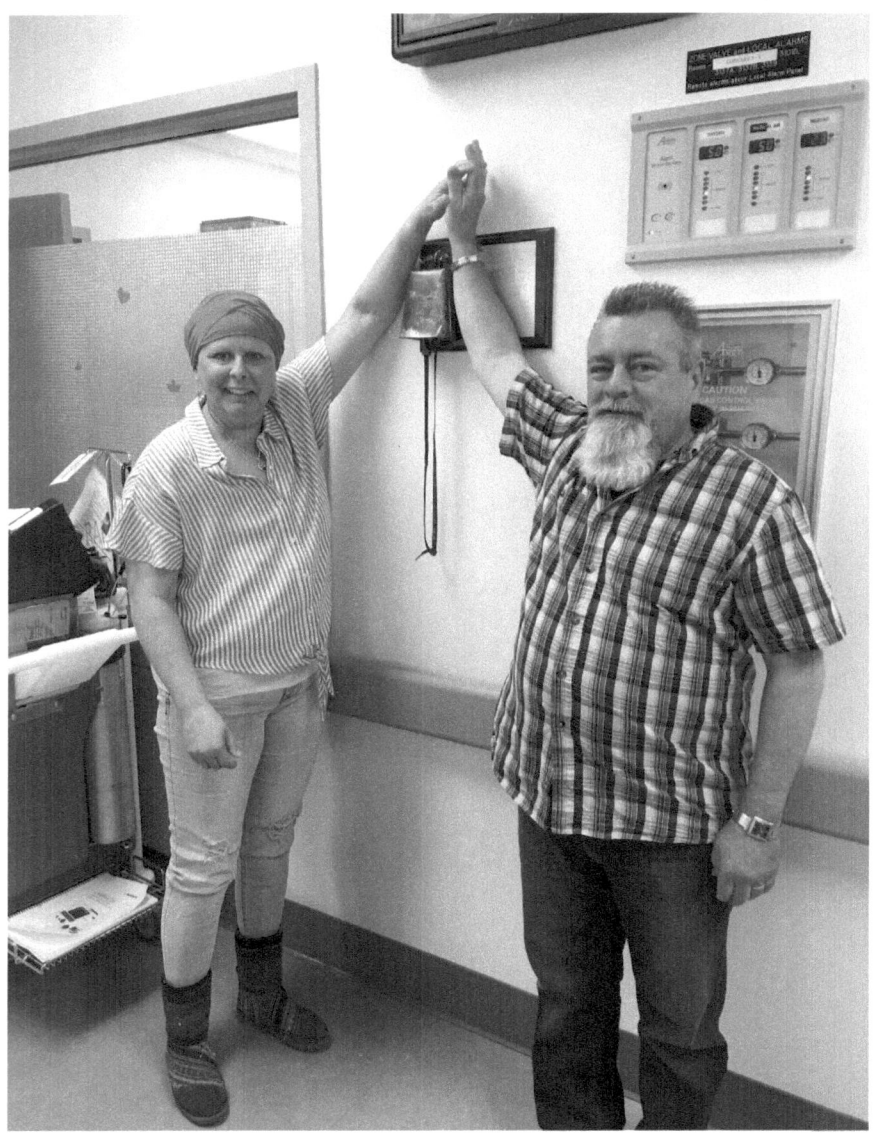

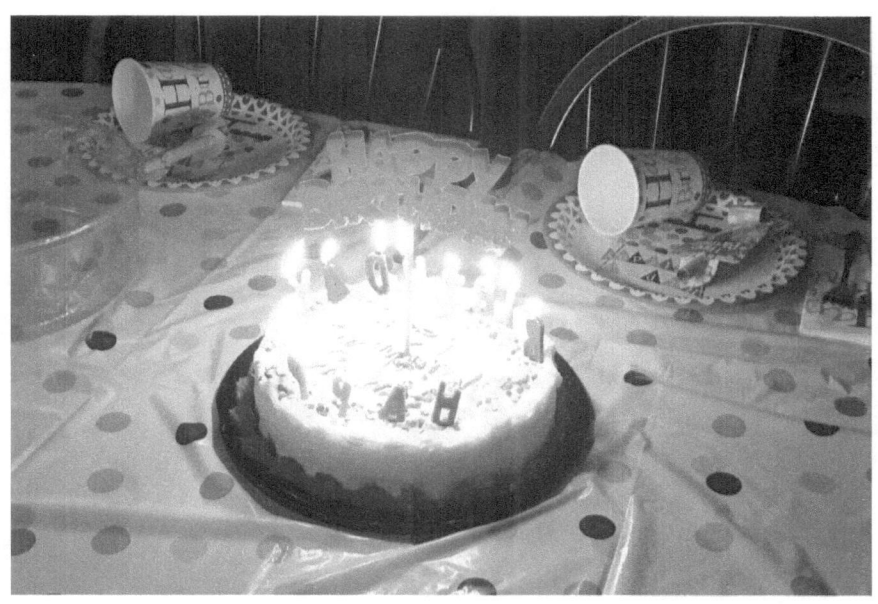

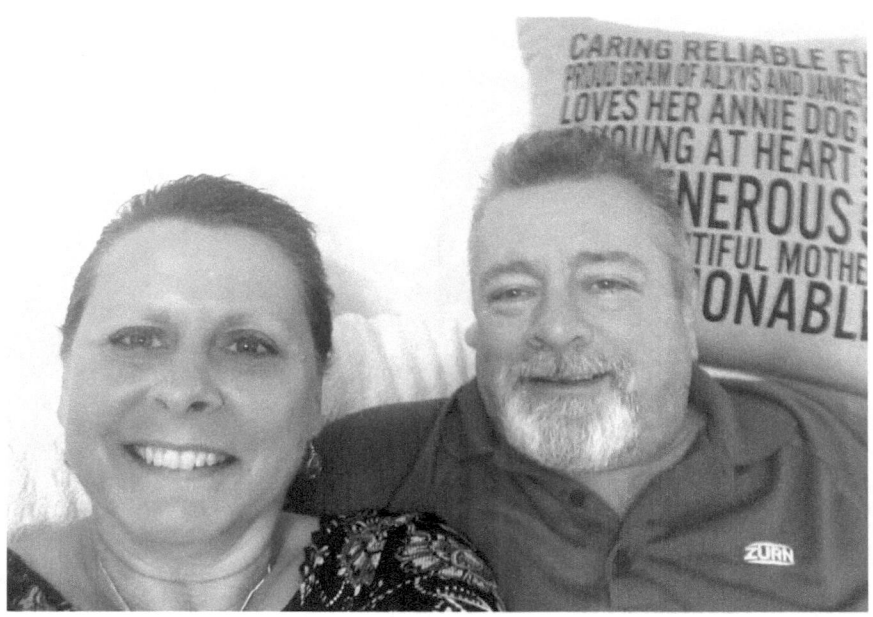

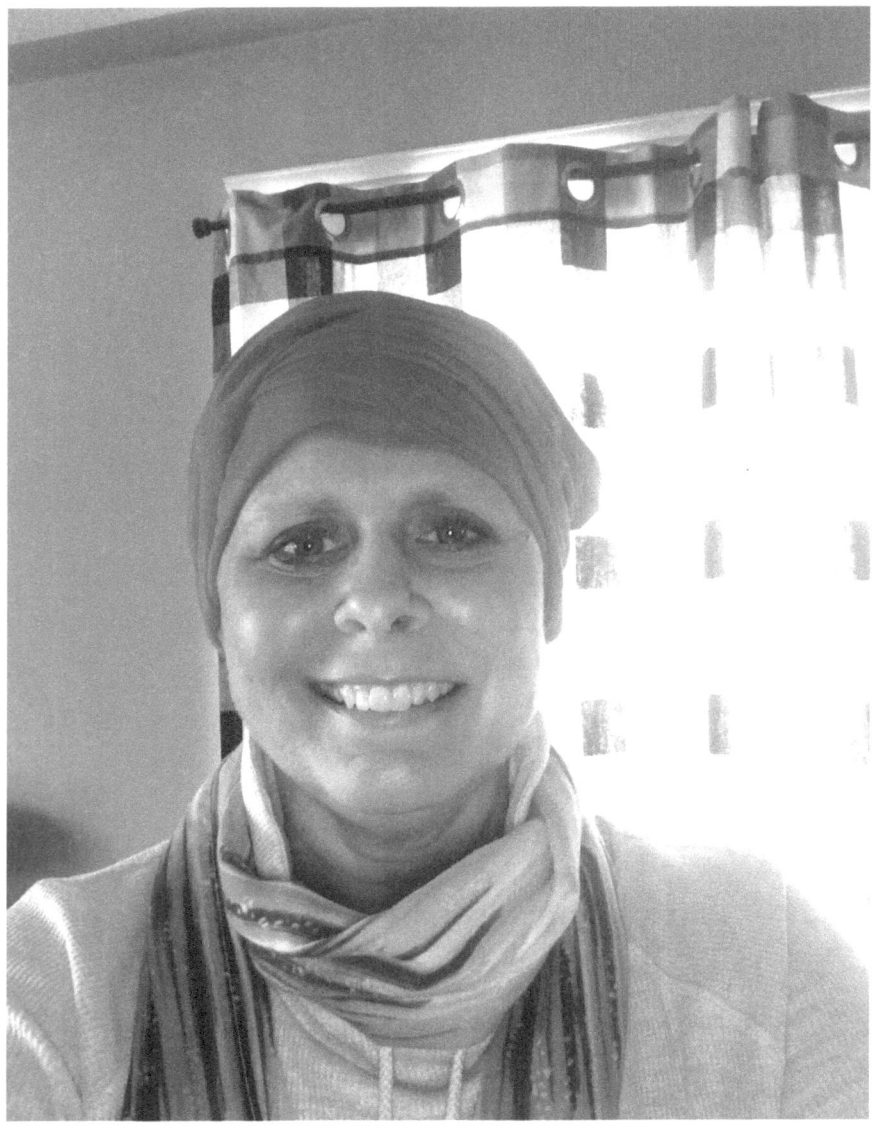

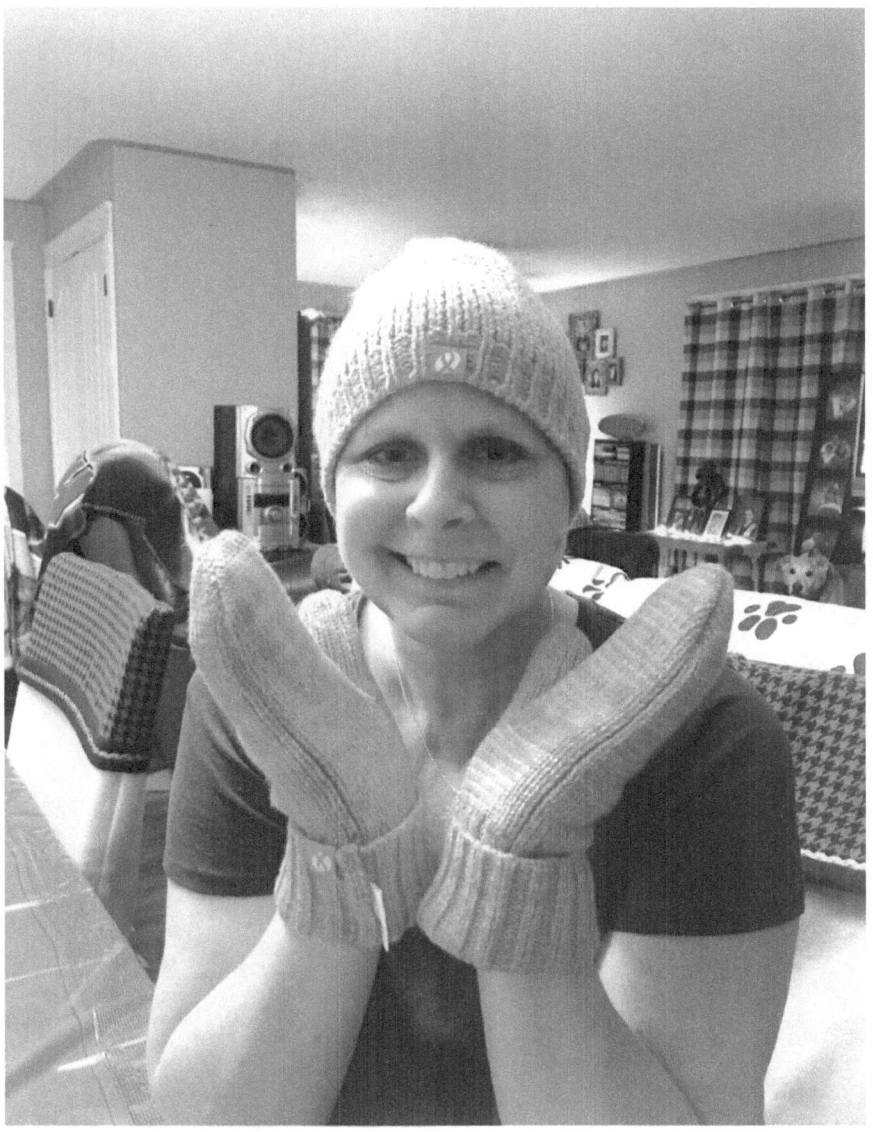

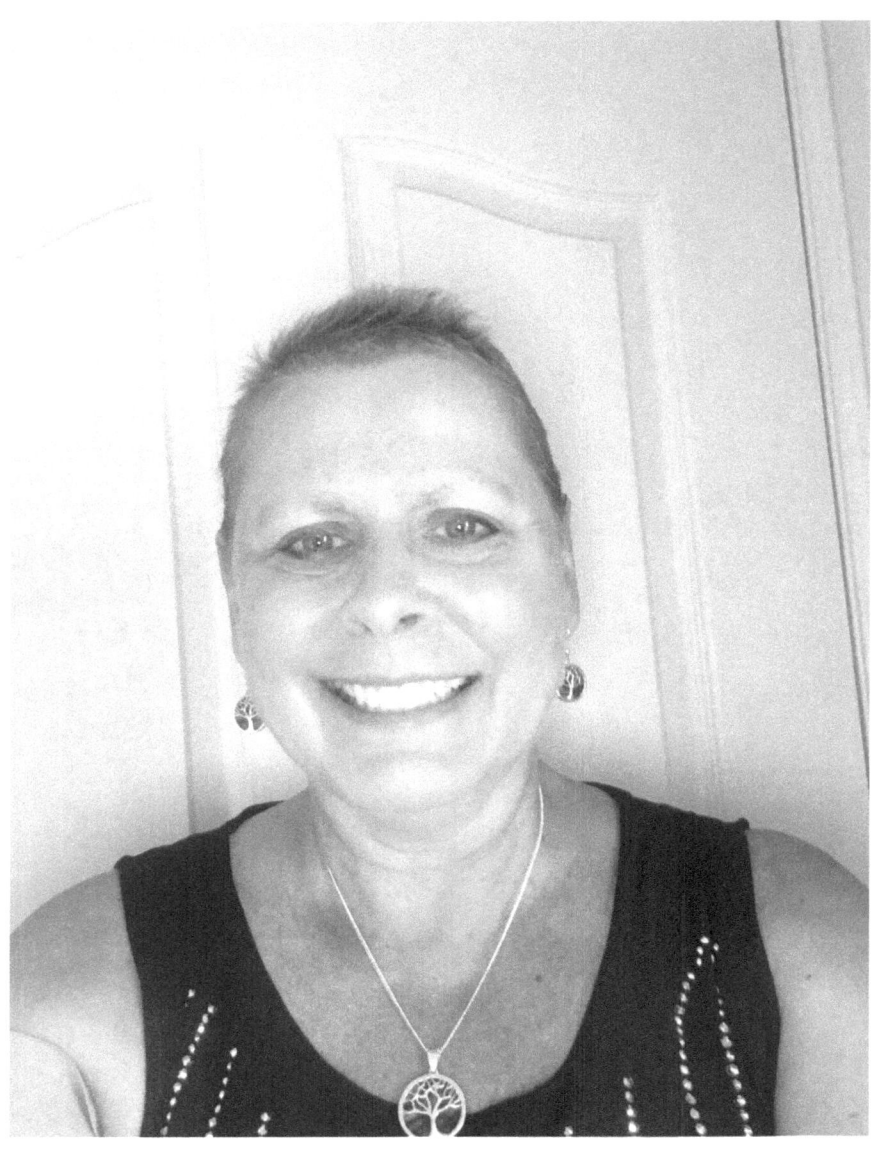

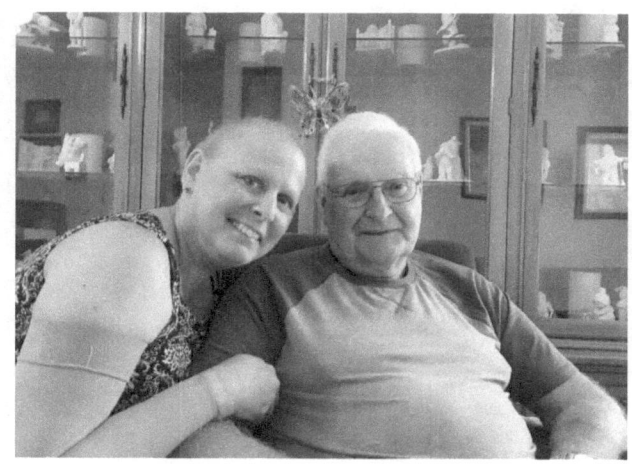

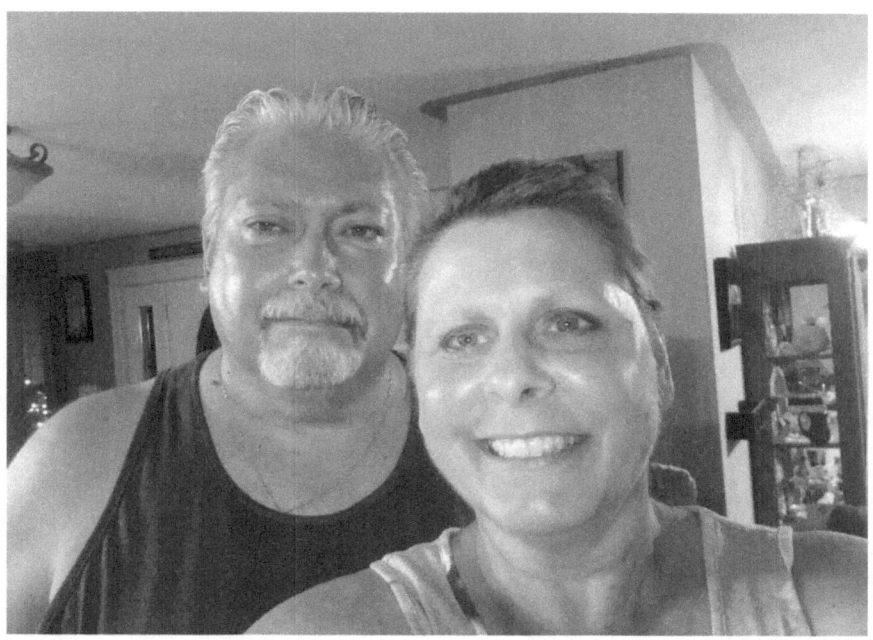

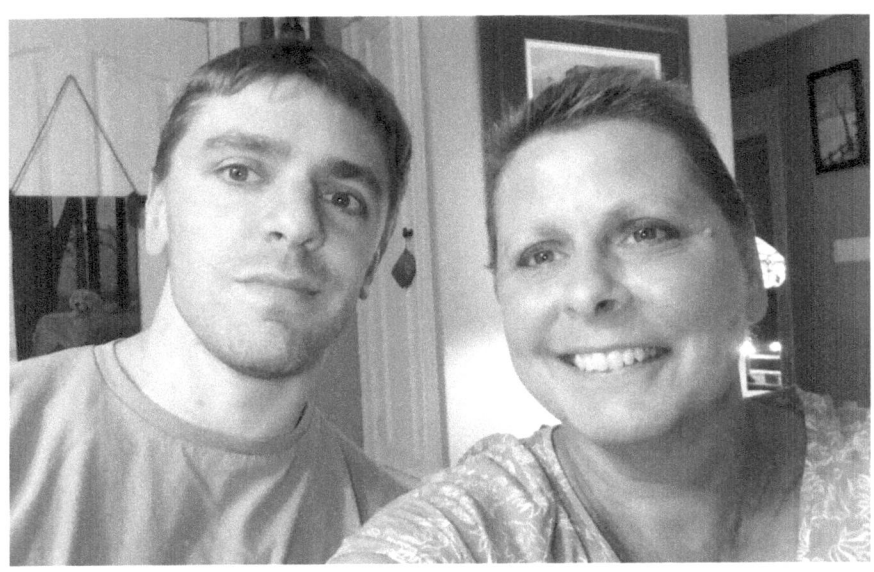

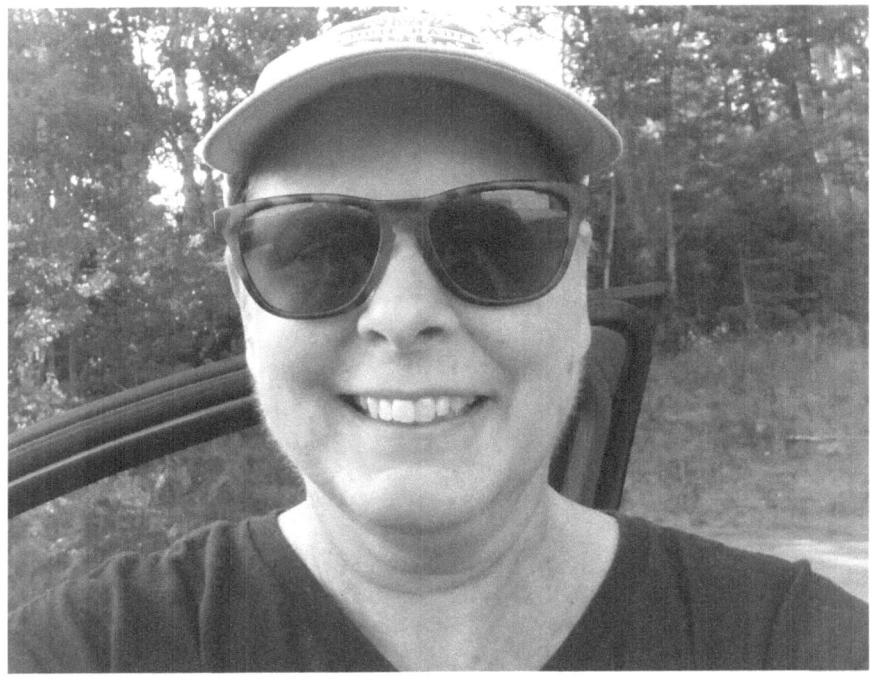

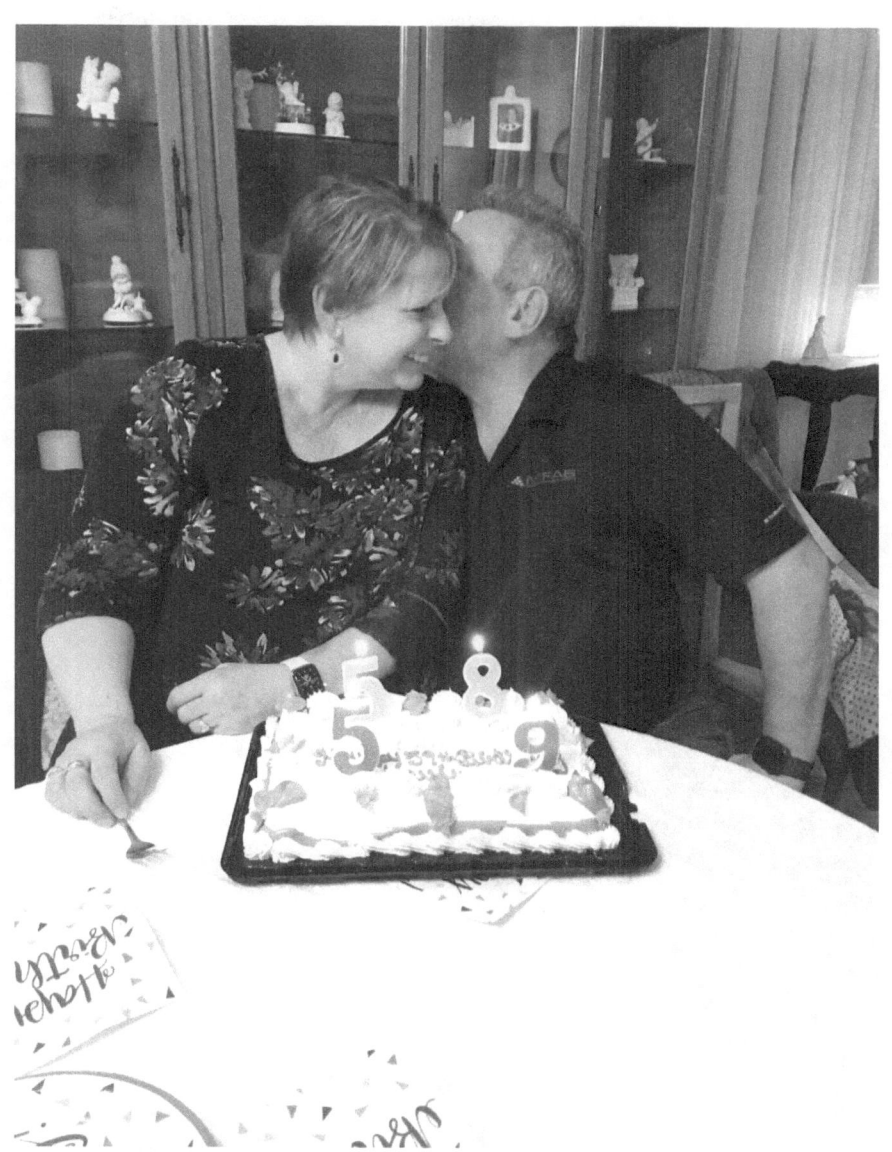

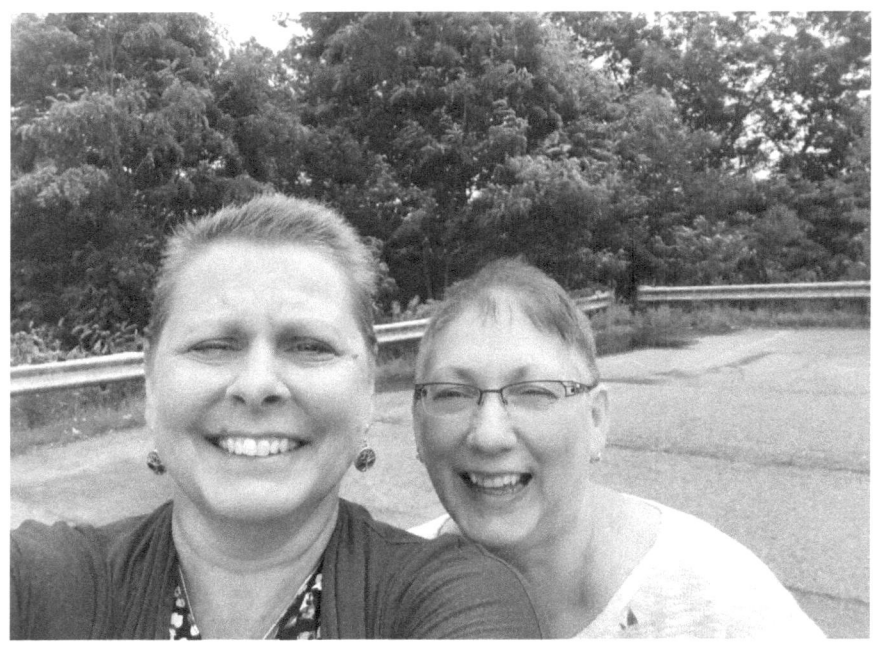

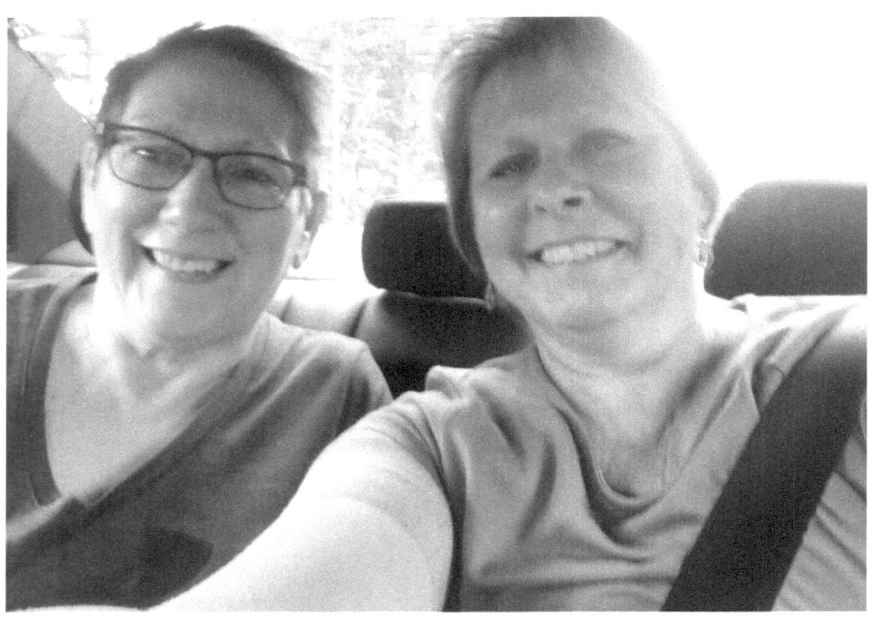

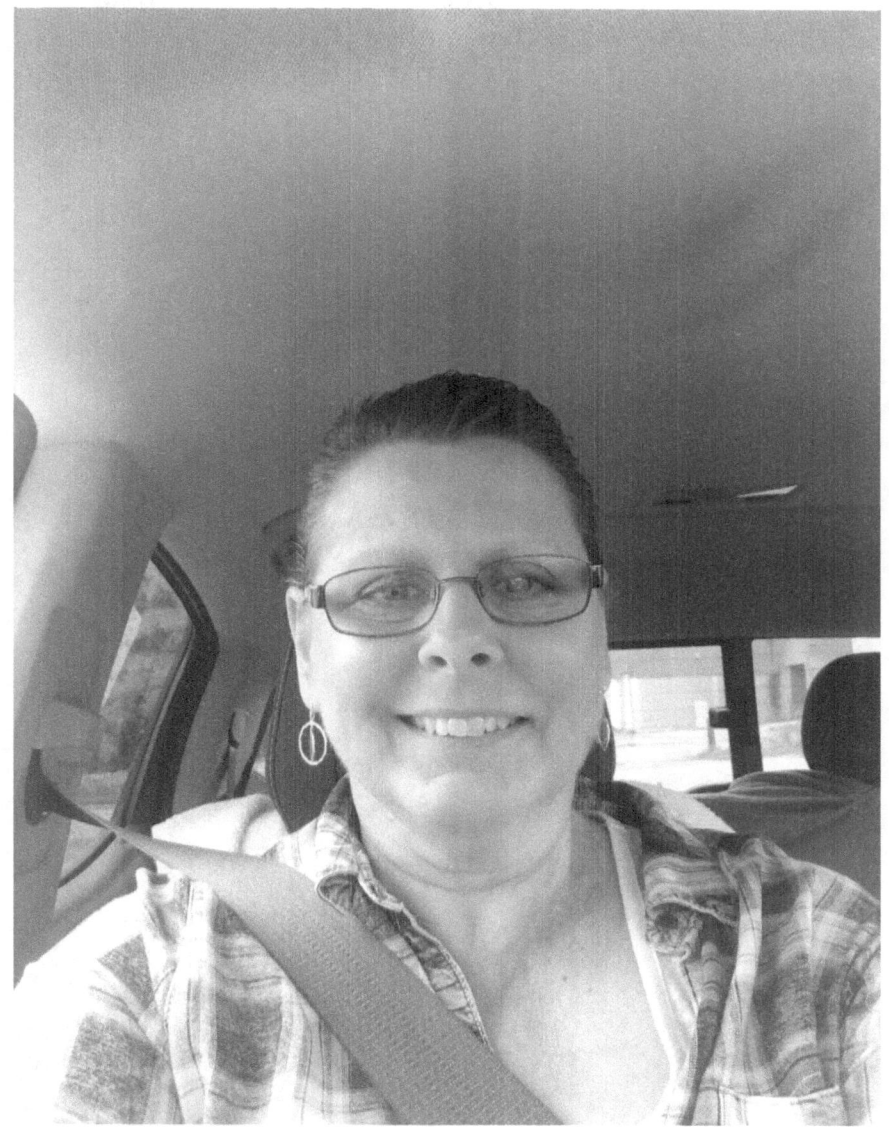

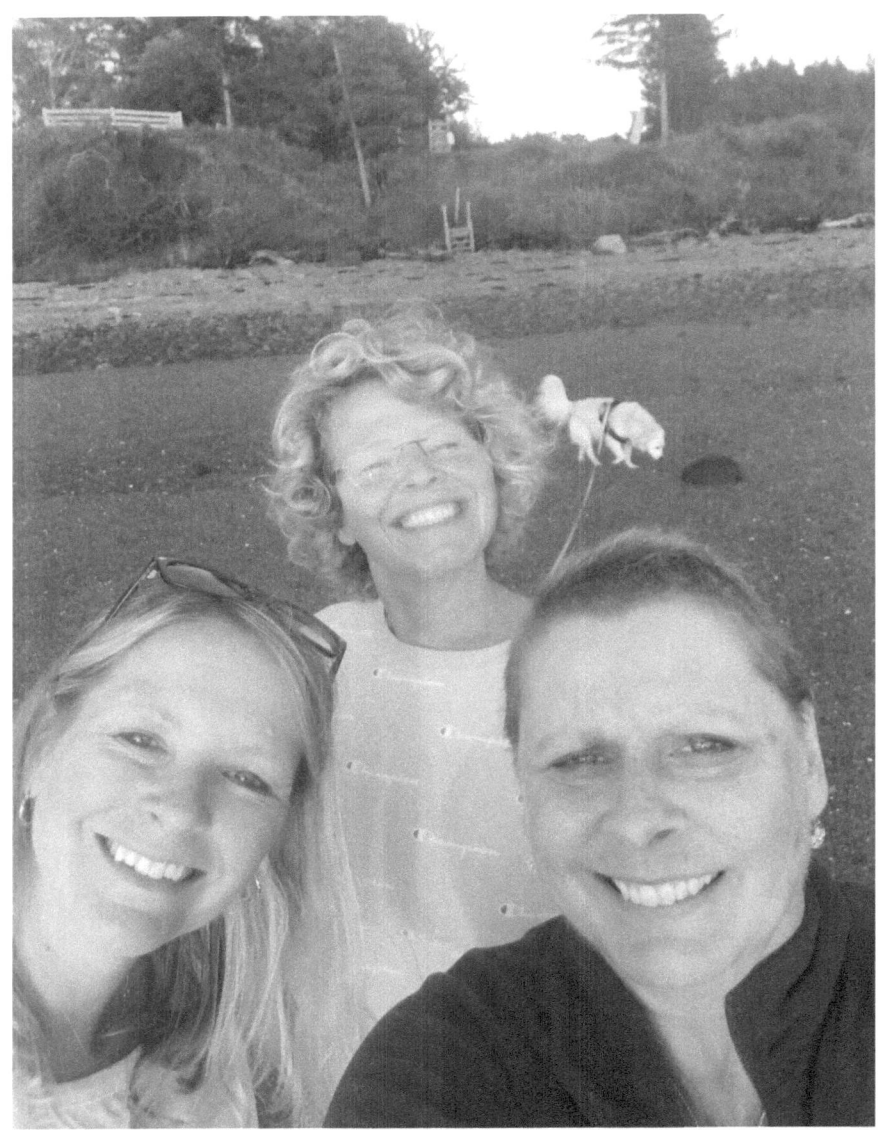

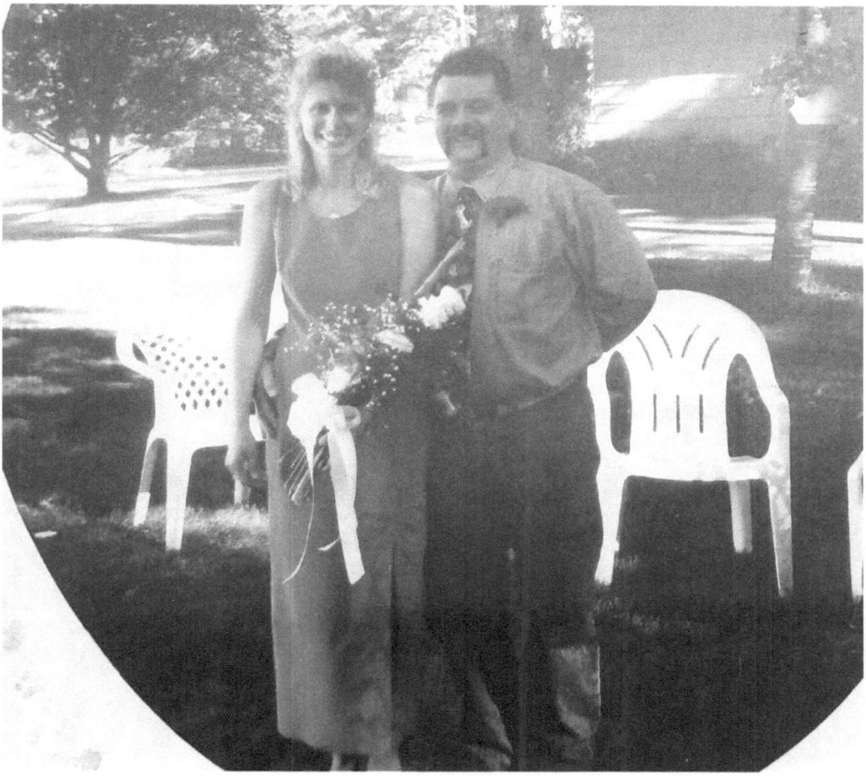

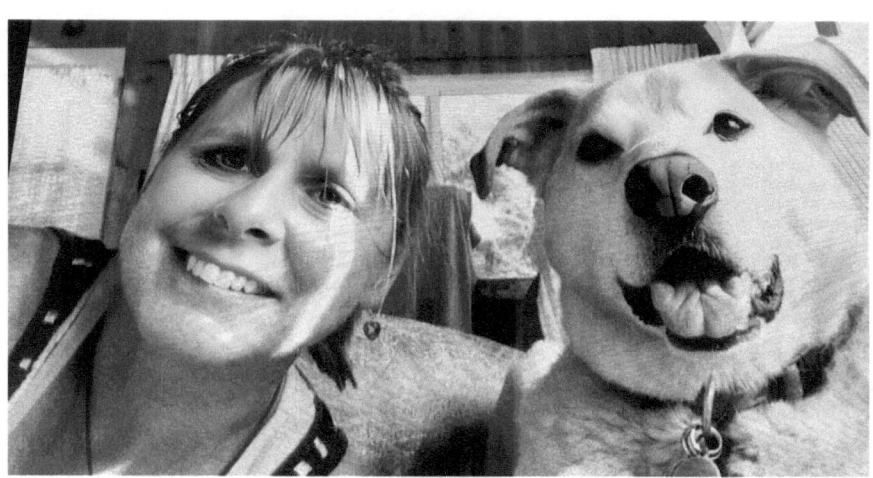

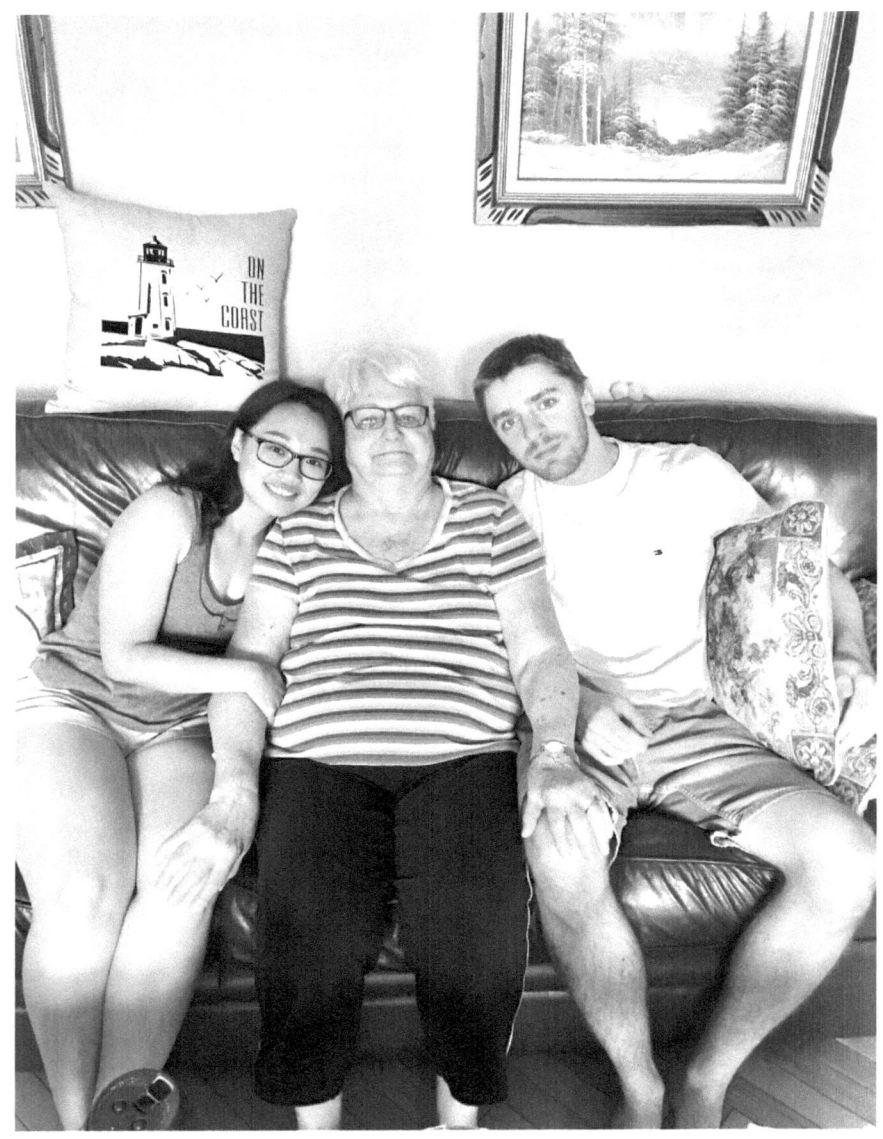

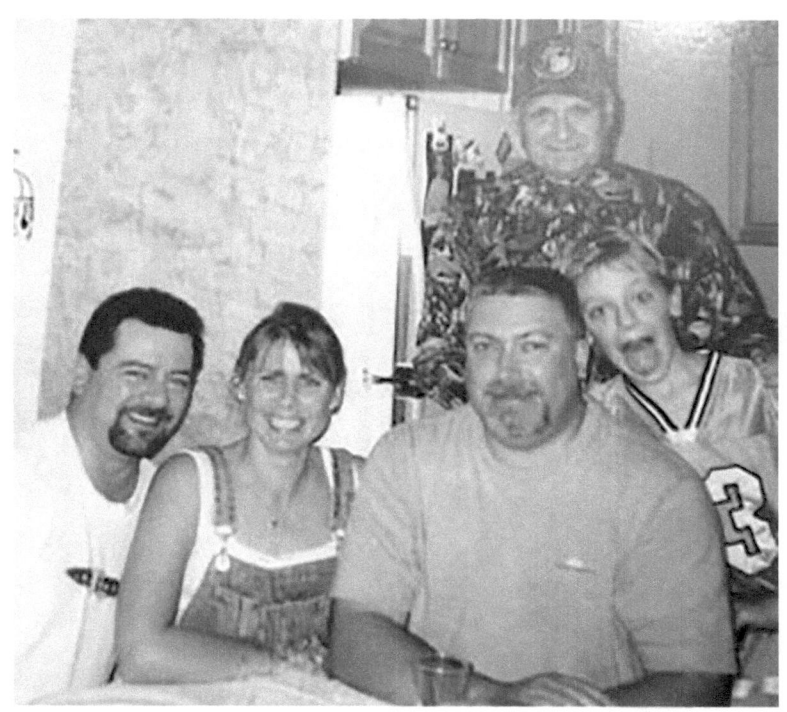

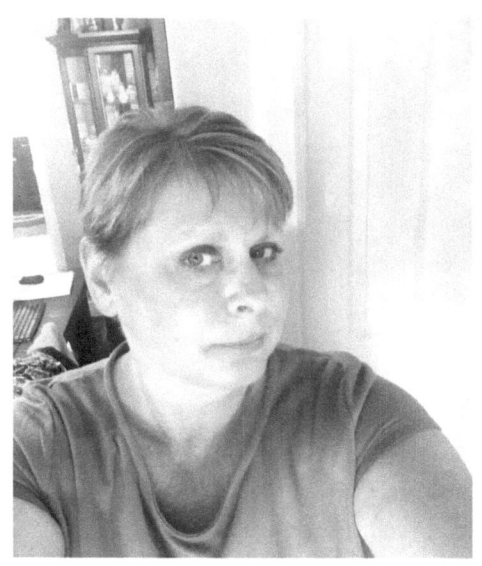

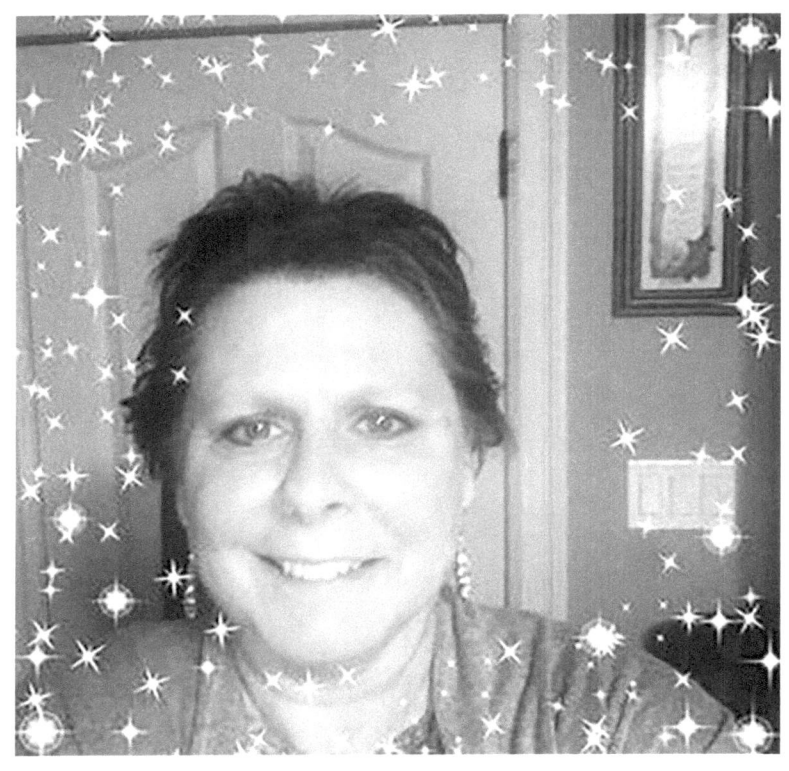

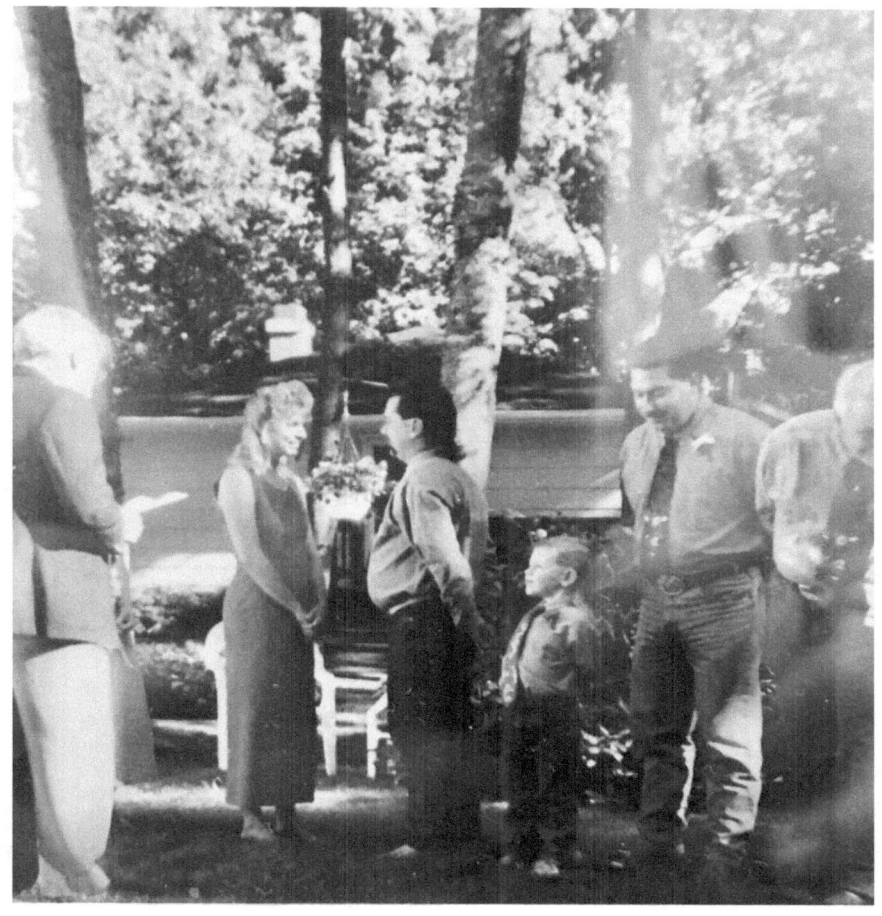

www.ingramcontent.com/pod-product-compliance
Lightning Source LLC
Chambersburg PA
CBHW051413280526
45785CB00003B/1049